THE
MICRODOSING
GUIDEBOOK

THE MICRODOSING GUIDEBOOK

A STEP-BY-STEP MANUAL TO IMPROVE YOUR PHYSICAL AND MENTAL HEALTH THROUGH PSYCHEDELIC MEDICINE

C. J. SPOTSWOOD, PMHNP

Published by:
Ulysses Press
PO Box 3440
Berkeley, CA 94703
www.ulyssespress.com

ISBN: 978-1-64604-310-1
Library of Congress Control Number: 2021946583

Printed in the United States by Kingery Printing Company
10 9 8 7 6 5 4 3 2

Acquisitions editor: Ashten Evans
Managing editor: Claire Chun
Editor: Scott Calamar
Proofreader: Renee Rutledge
Front cover design: Rebecca Lown
Interior design and layout: what!design @ whatweb.com
Production assistant: Yesenia Garcia Lopez
Artwork: cover—rainbow background © hunthomas/shutterstock.com, brain © Jolygon/shutterstock.com; interior—page 24 © chromatos/shutterstock.com, page 119 © VectorMine/shutterstock.com

IMPORTANT NOTE TO READERS: This book has been written and published for informational and educational purposes only. It is not intended to serve as medical advice or to be any form of medical treatment. You should always consult with your physician before altering or changing any aspect of your medical treatment. Do not stop or change any prescription medications without the guidance and advice of your physician. Any use of the information in this book is made on the reader's good judgment and is the reader's sole responsibility. This book is not intended to diagnose or treat any medical condition and is not a substitute for a physician. This book is independently authored and published and no sponsorship or endorsement of this book by, and no affiliation with, any trademarked brands or other products mentioned within is claimed or suggested. All trademarks that appear in this book belong to their respective owners and are used here for informational purposes only. The author and publisher encourage readers to patronize the brands mentioned in this book.

This book is dedicated to my friends, family, and mentors who have supported me along the road to publication and all of my personal journeys. I would also like to dedicate this book to all of my current and former patients. Without learning from you, writing it wouldn't have been possible.

CONTENTS

AUTHOR'S NOTE

This book is about ingesting very small doses of LSD or psilocybin with the aim of improving various areas of one's life without experiencing a full-on psychedelic effect.

I ask the reader to consider all of the following cautions before using any of the information in my book.

PSYCHEDELICS USED IN MICRODOSING. My book is limited to the use of LSD and psilocybin in microdosing. At no point am I referring to the use of ibogaine, ayahuasca, MDMA, or any other substances.

POSSIBLE POSITIVE HEALTH EFFECTS. Microdosers have reported experiencing improvements in their mental and physical health, focus, creativity, and spiritual awareness. However, medical research has not shown that microdosing psychedelic substances is more effective than a placebo for any medical or mental health application. I am in no way saying that microdosing is a panacea for all illnesses or conditions, or that every user will experience positive health effects.

POSSIBLE NEGATIVE HEALTH EFFECTS. The use of psyche-delics may result in negative health effects, and so does the discontinuation of medicines that you may be taking now. Some of the potential side effects, risks, and drug interactions are discussed in detail in Chapter 7 and Chapter 8. As noted below, you should discuss the health risks of microdosing—and the best way to reduce those risks—with your healthcare provider. Not doing so can result in serious consequences, including emotional and mental instability, discontinuation syndromes, increased suicidal thoughts, withdrawal symptoms, seizures, and even death.

CONSULT YOUR HEALTHCARE PROVIDER. Although I describe how psychedelics may interact with your health needs, including your medications, it is very important for you to consult your own primary care and/or psychiatric provider before using any psychedelics and *before* decreasing or stopping any medications that you may be using. The decision about whether or not to engage in microdosing is yours to make, but it depends on your own health issues. You should discuss the benefits and risks with a suitable healthcare provider before making a decision. See Chapter 11 for guidance on how to discuss microdosing with your healthcare provider.

LEGAL RISKS. One of the risks of microdosing is arrest and criminal prosecution. Psychedelics are categorized under federal law as Schedule I controlled substances, the most restrictive class of drugs, and they are defined as "drugs with no currently accepted medical use and a high potential for abuse." Some states and municipalities have "decriminalized" these substances for personal use, but that doesn't mean that they are entirely without legal consequences, including arrest and conviction for a crime. Before acquiring and/or using psychedelics, you must check with your local authorities—and consult an attorney—to determine what legal risks you are taking. The risk is even greater if you share these substances with others.

NO ENDORSEMENT. I have conducted extensive research for my book, and my sources are mentioned in the Acknowledgments and References. However, all of the opinions and advice in the book are mine alone, and no endorsement or affiliation with my sources is claimed or suggested.

GUIDING OTHERS. If you plan to use my book as a resource to help guide others, you should give all of these cautions to the people with whom you work.

INTRODUCTION

WHAT IS MICRODOSING AND WHY IS IT ALL THE RAGE?

Welcome! In recent years an increasing number of individuals have turned to psychedelic medicines, and the numbers seem to have risen further during the recent COVID-19 pandemic. While the use of high-dose psychedelics is evident, a growing number of people are interested in taking their health into their own hands through microdosing. Microdosing psychedelics is the act of ingesting subperceptual amounts of the substances with the aim of improving various areas of one's life—without experiencing a full-on psychedelic journey (aka tripping). For the purpose of this book, I focus only on psilocybin, LSD, or substances that have a similar structure to LSD. Microdosers have reported experiencing improvements in their mental and physical health, focus, creativity, and even spiritual awareness. It is believed that microdosing psychedelics has been practiced by indigenous cultures for centuries, from tribesmen in Mexico using peyote to hunters in the African Sahara Desert ingesting low doses of psilocybin to improve their visual acuity.

The act of microdosing psychedelics was relatively unknown until the release of *The Psychedelic Explorer's Guide* by James Fadiman in 2011. From there, word has grown, and we have seen various media outlets covering microdosing. These include *Rolling Stone*, the *Guardian*, *Playboy*, the *Economist*, *Forbes*, and even various major newspapers, including the *Washington Post* and the *New York Times*.

With all the talk out there about microdosing and its purported benefits, many have asked me, "How do I do it?" and "How do I find trusted information?" These questions provided the initial motivation for me to write this book. I didn't feel I could steer askers to a specific place that I could trust, nor did the answers I came across seem to have any significant scientific basis. The best information I could find is cited within the covers of this book. But even that information was incomplete or inconclusive, only provided in bits and pieces. That made it difficult to navigate the informational landscape, and there were no resources for a "how-to" approach. Here, I give readers full access to information in one place. Additionally, many of the online guides or books that I have read merely base their information on the author's or website owner's credibility, firsthand accounts, or anecdotal evidence. I'm not minimizing that information, but I wanted to know where it came from and took the opportunity to read it myself. I can say I have personally checked out and vetted any of the sources and information behind all the work cited within this book—we can't base everything on reputation. That being said, I want to point out that all the information provided within this guidebook comes from available published research. All I have done is read the research, synthesized the data, and disseminated the important information into one handy package.

THE MICRODOSING GUIDEBOOK

My approach to writing this guidebook is unique in that I will describe how psychedelics work, how they may interact with your unique health needs (including medications), and how to mitigate risks before you begin. You will also learn how microdosing may affect your holistic health, encompassing your physical, mental, emotional, and spiritual health needs. Additionally, I will provide information that may not directly be associated with microdosing but is relevant to improving health outcomes.

Surprisingly, when writing this book, I realized that not only are there no published guidebooks on how to microdose (to the best of my knowledge), but there aren't any resources readily available for medical professionals detailing the process of doing so. This guidebook is intended to bridge that gap. It is my hope that as you prepare to start a microdosing regimen, you will take this book with you to your next appointment with your primary care or psychiatric provider. Together, you can both decide if microdosing psychedelics may be right for you and collaboratively start a treatment plan. Part 2 of the handbook section is written specifically for healthcare providers. Here, I go more in-depth answering questions specific to them.

HOW TO USE THIS BOOK

This guidebook is divided into three sections. Part 1, "The Microdoser's Handbook," is for those who want to get up to speed on microdosing: how to do it, what conditions it may help, what its side effects are. Here you will learn how to come up with a plan–a protocol to follow–and how to find your optimal microdose. Part 2, "The Provider's Handbook," offers detailed medical and technical information aimed specifically at healthcare providers looking for information to support their patients. And finally, Part 3 offers a workbook to lead microdosers through the process, step by step, including journaling their experiences. This will help you incorporate your plan into your everyday life.

No matter if your intent behind getting this guidebook is strictly educational, in order to learn more about microdosing or how it may benefit you, or to use this as a resource to help guide others, I am glad that you have taken the first (or maybe next) step to understanding the benefits of microdosing psychedelics. There are many reasons one may want to microdose, but they all fit into one of three categories:

🌀 Improving performance: This includes improved creativity and focus; opening one's mind to new ways of seeing things; or finding creative new ways to solve problems.

🌀 Relieving pathological conditions: This includes both physical and mental health conditions such as depression, anxiety, pain, migraines, substance-use disorders, anorexia, and attention deficit hyperactivity disorder (ADHD), just to name a few. Many more conditions have been found to benefit from microdosing, many more are suspected, and potentially more applications haven't even been realized yet. I will discuss this in greater detail later in this guidebook. Additionally, I will explain why microdosing is different from conventional treatment methods.

🌀 Decreasing or stopping pharmaceuticals or drugs: Microdosing psychedelics can help one to come off various medications, often because microdosing's side effects are more tolerable or more effective. Some have incorporated microdosing into their sober-living plan, to break free of a chemical dependency.

I am in no way saying that microdosing is a panacea for all illnesses or conditions, but it may be an additional tool to provide the relief that the approaches of conventional medicine may not. As you will see ahead in the guidebook, the risk is low and the potential benefits high.

The point of this guidebook is not only to provide knowledge of how to safely engage in microdosing practices, but also to offer some tools to actively incorporate these practices into your everyday life. Many of the skills described within would be beneficial for anyone, regardless of if they are attempting to microdose, taking other forms of medication, or simply looking to make overall improvements in their life.

Unlike Western medicine's passive approach to physical and mental health, in which people often "take a pill and expect changes," it is my hope that you actively engage in your treatment. As with anything in life, the more you put into something, the more you gain from it, and active participation in any treatment improves clinical outcomes and satisfaction.

If you get stuck at any point when reading this guidebook, set it down, practice meditation, mindfulness, or one of the other skills gained within this book, and allow yourself time to focus on something other than the task at hand. Then come back later when you are ready. This guidebook is not meant to be overwhelming, nor is it set up to be read cover to cover. Read it as you would like, one section at a time, or jump around to areas that you feel are important to you. Remember, two great philosophies that come from psychedelic circles are relevant here:

🌀 The medicine will bring the answers (or questions) forward to reveal themselves.

🌀 "Doing by not doing." This is the idea that sometimes, not taking action can be productive in helping matters fall into place naturally.

PSILOCYBIN AND LSD

Psilocybin and LSD (or its derivatives) are the two most common substances used for microdosing. They have similar chemical structures, but LSD binds tighter to receptors, so it hits a little harder and lasts longer. I would like to note that Albert Hofmann, the first person to synthesize LSD, described it as being similar to an atom bomb, whereas psilocybin is a weapon of conventional strength. This, of course, refers to macro or large dosages, not microdoses as this guidebook describes.

HARM-REDUCTION MODEL

Since I have started writing and talking about the use of psychedelics as medicine, many have asked how I could speak about illegal substances in such a manner. My answer: I discuss the science, published literature, and how, in my opinion, they are wrongfully classified as Schedule I drugs since they obviously do have "medical value." I add that on a daily basis I educate my patients and their families about numerous drugs, both legal and illegal, emphasizing that if they choose to use those drugs, they should do so as safely as possible. This is what is known as the "harm-reduction model," which I used as the basis for this book and the motivations behind it. If people are going to take psychedelics, both macro and microdoses, they should be aware of the risks, benefits, and how to approach their use in the safest way possible. However, while the harm-reduction model is better known, this book comes more from a "risk-reduction" model. Some may use the words "harm" and "risk" interchangeably or say this word choice is a matter of semantics, but I think it is important to differentiate the two.

"Harm reduction" infers these substances may have an inherent harm to taking them. Research has shown over and over that these substances are not harmful when taken in a safe and thought-out manner, but they do have some inherent risks. Many of the risks can be mitigated through careful planning and collaborative work between individuals and their healthcare team. For these reasons, I think it is important to start using risk reduction as opposed to harm reduction; if nothing else it may help to decrease the stigma and negative connotation associated with psychedelics. Maybe, by changing these preconceived notions, we can start to see these substances shift culturally from "drugs" to their more proper place as "medicines."

Admittedly, and to much of the chagrin of microdosing advocates, modern research has not shown microdosing psychedelic medicines to be more effective than placebo for any medical or mental health applications. This guidebook provides strong evidence showing the theoretical mechanisms of the actions of microdosing, theories behind their application, and the most up-to-date research supporting the use of microdosing psychedelics as medicine. In addition, when research is lacking, I use what is available, ranging from peer-reviewed publications to books to websites. Often, what is published describes what is known regarding *macro*doses of psychedelics, not *micro*doses. In these cases, I attempt to extrapolate hypothetical conclusions and describe how I came to my conclusions.

I've presented the information in this book as clearly and efficiently as possible in order to provide you with the safest approach. I have taken all efforts to include as many special circumstances as I could, which means potentially taking a polypharmaceutical approach—this all too often occurs in medicine, especially concerning mental health. Research has shown that some medications don't have any potential interactions with psychedelics while other medications do. These interactions' responses vary from minor to major to fully blocking all the potential benefits microdosing offers.

I want to be clear I am *not* "anti-medication" by any means. I prescribe many of the medications described in this guidebook and understand that medications are necessary for many individuals. I know those who report how medications were life changing for them, as well as those who have stopped their medications for various reasons, including experiencing intolerable side effects. Microdosing may be life changing for some, who tolerate it better than conventional approaches. But please, please, please consult with your healthcare provider before you begin this program and if you intend to make any medication changes. Not doing so can result in serious consequences, including emotional and mental instability, discontinuation syndromes, increased suicidal thoughts, withdrawal syndromes, seizures, and even death. Having a frank and open discussion with your healthcare provider, then collaboratively making a plan to discontinue or taper medications, must be done ahead of time as a safer option (and to better tolerate the microdosing regimen).

One major point to note: At no point in this guidebook am I referring to the use of ibogaine, ayahuasca, or MDMA as the medicine to microdose. The presence of monoamine oxidase inhibitors (MAOIs) in the ayahuasca brew and ibogaine/ MDMA's serotonin reuptake actions (along with its effects on opiate receptors) make these substances completely different from those of the "classical psychedelics," thus putting them outside the scope of this book.

Once again, welcome to *The Microdosing Guidebook*. I am excited to guide you on your journey and wish you the best of luck.

Mush love and namaste,

C. J.

PART 1:
THE MICRODOSER'S HANDBOOK

CHAPTER 1

WHAT IS PSILOCYBIN, AND HOW MIGHT IT HELP ME?

Psilocybin (4-phosphoryloxy-N,N-dimethyltryptamine) is a naturally occurring psychedelic prodrug of the tryptamine family, and it is found in over two hundred different species of mushrooms all around the world. Some of the most common come from the genus *Psilocybe*. Psilocybin is referred to as a "prodrug" because in order for it to become active, it must be converted to psilocin, the active chemical that is responsible for its psychoactive effects, in the intestinal tract through a process of dephosphorylation. Since psilocybin is a prodrug, injecting it (or injecting psilocybin tea) will not result in psychedelic effects. It will make you sick and could result in death. You may notice in some academic studies that the researchers administered IV (intravenous) infusions. This is psilocin, not psilocybin. For the purpose of this guidebook, I will simply refer to it as psilocybin and the route of administration is intended to be by mouth.

Both psilocybin's and lysergic acid diethylamide's (LSD) primary mechanisms of action are through agonism (activation) of serotonin receptors found throughout the body, most notably the serotonin 5-HT2A receptors. This is further discussed later in this guidebook, but for now, check out the chemical structure of LSD, psilocin, and serotonin. Notice anything? Look at how chemically similar they appear to be.

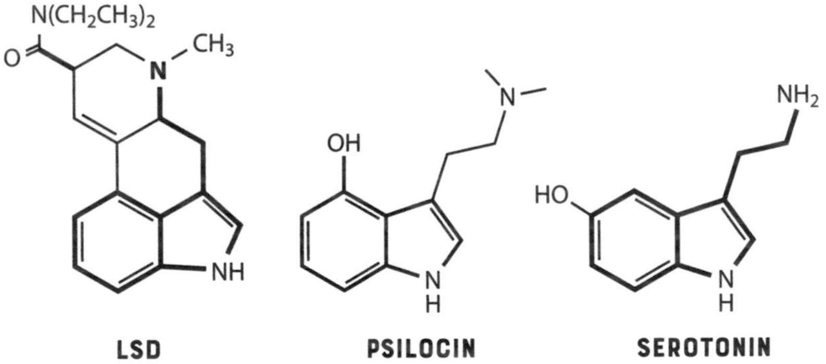

Figure 1: Chemical structures of LSD, psilocin, and serotonin.

Psilocybes also have other hallucinogenic chemicals within the mushroom, which at this point are less understood by researchers. The exact amount varies depending on the specific species of psilocybe. Some of these chemicals include, but are not limited to: baeocystin, norbaeocystin, norpsilocin, bufotenin, and aeruginascin. There may be more that have yet to be identified. These other chemicals are beyond the scope of this book, and I will focus mostly on psilocybin/psilocin.

Why should we take these other chemicals into consideration? As mentioned, at this point we don't fully understand what these chemicals are or what they do in the body, but they may be important. Much of the current research is being conducted with pure psilocin, not the actual fungi/fruit body. In the pure form, the psilocybin has been converted to psilocin before administration, so the body doesn't need to do the work to achieve effect. With this process, the other chemicals are stripped out of the medicine, leaving only psilocin. But these other chemicals may contribute to the healing properties of psilocybin as part of the "entourage effect." The entourage effect is the theory that numerous compounds can act together synergistically to enhance the overall effect. Think of it as your favorite band: Have you ever listened to them in their solo efforts and felt like something was just missing? It was. You're missing how the band as a whole brings out the best in each other. This may be one of the drawbacks of researchers using pure substances as opposed to naturally occurring fungi. This is one of my biggest fears/concerns when it comes to big pharma/big money getting involved in the psychedelic space, but I digress.

In some studies comparing the full fruit/fungi (with the other chemicals still present) to pure extracted psilocin, the full fungi sample was more effective in reducing anxious behaviors in rats (Matsushima et al. 2009). Additionally, the full fungi were found to be ten times more effective in changing behavioral responses in rats (Zhuk et al. 2015). To compare, how often have you read about marijuana's therapeutic benefits? Those benefits are attributed to not just THC, but also to the nonpsychoactive substance CBD. This may have been why the pharmaceutical Marinol (dronabinol), a synthetic marijuana, was found by many to be less effective than plant and plant extracts. I feel we should be mindful of these other chemicals for future research and keep them in the back of our minds as we start to see more technological advances and patents in the field of psychedelic medicines. Hopefully, one day we will understand these chemicals better, but for now, the potential of the entourage effect is one reason why I am a proponent of the plant-based medicine movement versus the medicalization models we are seeing.

The research is clear that substantial physical and neurochemical changes are brought about by high-dose psychedelics. Significant research has been conducted over the years showing how to take these changes and utilize them in clinical applications, but we aren't completely there yet. Theories are still evolving on what exactly is happening neurochemically in the brain and why high-dose psychedelics elicit change. In addition, new hypothetical applications continue to be explored. At this point, we are not entirely sure what occurs at lower, subperceptual or microdoses, both physically and psychologically. It is for this reason much of the information in this guidebook is theoretical and exploratory. It is my hope that I clearly describe the science behind what we do know and how people have come to these theoretical conclusions.

HISTORY OF MICRODOSING PSYCHEDELICS

The concept of microdosing psychedelics is not new. Many believe that microdosing has been practiced by indigenous cultures for centuries for different reasons. Outside of these indigenous practices, Western medicine's fascination with psychedelics didn't begin until the late 1950s, when chemist Albert Hofmann and his employer Sandoz Laboratories were able to produce and distribute their newest medications, Indocybin and Delysid. These medications were nothing more than medical-grade synthetic psilocybin and LSD, respectively.

At that time, Indocybin (synthetic psilocybin) was used to help facilitate psychotherapeutic sessions, while Delysid (LSD) was touted as a panacea for all psychiatric ailments, and Sandoz even encouraged both psychiatrists and their students to use the LSD in order to gain a unique understanding of their patients who were diagnosed with schizophrenia. Sandoz, which felt that LSD was so revolutionary, made their LSD readily available to researchers around the world—for free. The smallest dosage available at that time, in tablets or ampules, was 25 mcg, what we would now consider as being at the higher end of a microdose.

In 2019, psychiatrist and psychedelic researcher Dr. Torsten Passie released *The Science of Microdosing Psychedelics*, which for the first time ever shed light on the mystery of microdosing psychedelics and microdosing's early research. Until that time, there had been evidence that Sandoz researched applications for microdosing their psychedelic medicines. In researching his book, Passie found letters by the late professor Hanscarl Leuner (1921–1996), a psycholytic therapist who also worked with hallucinogenic substances, describing how Sandoz employees had delivered psilocybin to him. In these letters there were descriptions of high-dose psilocybin and LSD necessary for inducing states of depersonalization for psychotherapy, but there was also mention of smaller, even microdosing, amounts he was exploring.

In his 2019 book, Passie described how researchers had hoped to be able to use low-dose psychedelics to reduce obsessional-compulsive symptoms and anxiety in participants. Passie quoted the authors, stating, "It is too early to definitely judge the efficacy of psilocybin. But at least there have been some quite remarkable successes seen with treatment" (Augsberger 1959, 2). Passie explains that while it was unclear if Sandoz expanded this research further and what those results may have been, he is aware of others who conducted similar experiments and reported similar positive results.

Lastly, in *The Science of Microdosing Psychedelics*, Passie described numerous early LSD projects focusing on low or microdose amounts of LSD. Often these projects "proved" inconclusive effects or found respondents did not experience measurable effects when dosages were below 25 micrograms (we will use "mcg," but you may also see the symbol µg in some literature). In retrospect, I suspect that many of the researchers may have found respondents did not experience any notable psychedelic effects. Perhaps participants did not exhibit any obvious or measurable effects, or researchers were not attuned to the effects the microdoses were producing. For this reason, I am a strong proponent for reproducing some of the early psychedelic research with modern standards and technology.

The concept of microdosing psychedelics is discussed in early psychedelic literature, often for various psychotherapeutic applications. One such example, as described in one of the earliest manuals for psychedelic psychotherapy, the *Handbook for the Therapeutic Use of LSD: Individual and Group Procedures* (Blewett and Chewlos 1959), describes how administration of microdoses to some participants in high-dose psychedelic psychotherapy sessions allowed the participants to work "in close empathy" with others within the structure of the psychotherapy session. Those participants who received the microdoses either may be other patients within the group receiving psychotherapy and/or co-therapists facilitating the psychotherapy session. I want to note, if you were not aware, that during this period of psychedelic exploration, it was common for group facilitators to ingest psychedelics with their clients for their sessions, some even ingesting high-dose, fully psychedelic amounts of medicines.

It was believed that all participants ingesting psychedelics in the group setting, even at low doses, would foster a sense of closeness and elicit more empathetic responses from participants. These subperceptual dosages would maintain the participants' ability to interact and respond to others, while still remaining free from cognitive and sensory alterations. Some, such as Dr. Stanislav Grof, author of the psychedelic psychotherapy manual *LSD Psychotherapy* (1980) and the world's most experienced psychedelic psychotherapist (having led over five thousand sessions in his lifetime), felt that low-dose psychedelics had other, more mystical properties. Grof asserted that subperceptual doses of psychedelics would allow individuals the ability to interact in a subconscious or unconscious manner, even going so far as to allude those participants acquired the ability to communicate telepathically with others within the group setting. These abilities would not be achieved without first ingesting psychedelic substances, even if the effects were subperceptual.

I know some of these concepts seem far-fetched, even downright unbelievable by today's standards, but we should at least consider how it is almost impossible to study or research these theories. Maybe it is something we should at least consider: the concept, after all, is not too dissimilar to Paul Stamets' proposed mycological network, which connects all living beings on the earth.

Most of the early low-dose psychedelic research was funded by the US federal government, and their findings were more scientifically based, when compared to the hypothetical group-therapy applications. This research included gaining an understanding of LSD's subjective and physiological threshold and establishing dosage-dependent responses from participants. After these factors were better understood, the federal government began exploring various applications for the military and the CIA.

Many of these projects were small-scale applications, such as attempting to find ways to force agent interrogations, akin to a "truth serum," or efforts to improve soldiers' performance. Unfortunately, most of these results were inconclusive or lost over time. A double-blind placebo study that was not lost had tested soldiers' performance playing speed chess. The results noted a small loss in skill by participants, which is aligned with results in similar studies that are more recent.

Meanwhile, the US government explored other, larger-scale applications, with more nefarious intentions. The best known was the US government's hope to use low dosages of psychedelics as a chemical warfare agent, attempting to afflict numerous individuals at once via the community water supply.

Outside of the hypothetical applications of low-dose psychedelics buried within psychedelic psychotherapeutic handbooks, or the brief mentions about the US government's failed attempts to produce super soldiers or the next Manchurian Candidate, the idea of low-dose or microdoses of psychedelics was virtually unknown outside of the psychedelic community. There are reports in which former psychedelic researchers and their friends discussed the potential for microdoses, but often these ideas were not shared with outsiders, though those in the know were aware. This is until James Fadiman released *The Psychedelic Explorer's Guide* in 2011.

One notable exception where the concept of microdosing was mentioned briefly but specifically was in an interview with Albert Hofmann, the man who discovered LSD, in *High Times* magazine. Asked if there were any general medical uses for LSD to be marketed in the future, Hoffman replied "Very small doses, perhaps 25 micrograms, could be useful as a euphoriant or antidepressant" (Horowitz 1976).

I would also encourage you to explore some other mentions of microdosing discussed in Passie's 2019 *The Science of Microdosing Psychedelics*.

CHAPTER 2

PSYCHEDELICS AND PSYCHIATRY... A MATCH MADE IN HEAVEN?

Many people remember vaguely that LSD and other psychedelic drugs were once used experimentally in psychiatry, but few realize how much and how long they were used. This was not a quickly rejected and forgotten fad. Between 1950 and the mid-1960s there were more than a thousand clinical papers discussing 40,000 patients, several dozen books, and six international conferences on psychedelic drug therapy. It aroused the interest of many psychiatrists who were in no sense cultural rebels or especially radical in their attitudes.

—Grinspoon and Bakalar, *Psychedelic Drugs Reconsidered*

Many believe that we are currently in uncharted waters in regard to the use of psychedelic substances for the treatment of mental health disorders. This couldn't be further from the truth.

There is no doubt that psychedelics have helped to change the world to what we know it to be today, and I'm not just talking about what they did to music and culture in the 1960s.[1] One could even argue the discovery of neurochemistry, namely serotonin, and many of the treatments for mental health disorders such as depression and anxiety, are a direct result of the accidental (or the serendipitous) discovery of LSD by Albert Hofmann in 1943. After the discovery of LSD, it was ten years until serotonin was discovered in the mammalian brain. Then, a year later, in 1954, Woolley and Shaw described how "mental disturbances caused by lysergic acid diethylamide were to be attributed to an interference with the action of serotonin in the brain (Woolley and Shaw 1954, 229)." Without psychedelics, who knows how long it would have been before we started to understand what serotonin is. Even today, we still don't fully understand serotonin's role or actions, which I'll explore throughout this guidebook.

If anything, we are now in a psychedelic renaissance, attempting to make up for the lost time and lost research that resulted from Nixon's war on drugs in the late 1960s. According to the US Drug Enforcement Administration (DEA), classical psychedelics (and even marijuana) are classified as Schedule I controlled substances, the highest classification, reserved for substances that do not have any medical value and are highly addictive. Unfortunately, when psychedelic substances became

1.   To learn more about psychedelia and how it influenced culture in the 1960s, check out *American Trip* by Ido Hartogsohn.

scheduled by the FDA, not only did it limit access for individuals, but it also halted progress for researchers and clinicians who were successfully using psychedelics in therapeutic settings. Many had lofty goals and aspirations, hoping to learn more about these sacred, misunderstood substances, and attempting to find ways to apply their awesome properties. One of these individuals, Dr. Steven Pollock, aspired to one day open his own mycological research and treatment center. Who knows what we may have learned if it hadn't been for his murder in 1981.[2] Now, we are left with only a glimpse into his thoughts and ideas of how mushrooms would one day change the world. In hindsight, he was in many ways correct, and we are only now finding ways to utilize these psychedelic substances for various medical applications, probably much to the chagrin of federal officials.

Contrary to popular belief, no statistically significant association exists between psychedelic use and increased rates of serious psychological issues such as depression, anxiety, or suicidal thoughts (Johansen and Krebs 2015). In fact, users of psychedelic substances have been found to have lower rates of psychological distress overall, and previous users have lower rates of both inpatient hospitalizations and prescription medication use for mental health conditions across their lifespan (Krebs and Johansen 2013). Individuals who have used psychedelics even seem to have better overall physical health (Simonsson, Sexton, and Hendricks 2021).

At this point, the causes of many psychiatric conditions are not completely understood. Effective treatments for many medical

---

2. To learn more about the controversy surrounding the murder of Dr. Pollock, I encourage you to read "Blood Spore" by Hamilton Morris (https://harpers.org/archive/2013/07/blood-spore).

and psychiatric conditions have proven themselves to be quite challenging. The currently accepted psychopharmacological treatment modalities are in many ways inadequate and downright ineffective for many. The current pharmacological approaches to psychiatric care are merely palliative attempts to address symptoms, not really "curing" the underlying condition or diagnosis. For many, they are unable to achieve the complete eradication of numerous mental health symptoms, and improvements are often temporary, with symptoms returning once the individual stops taking the medication.

Maybe the most frustrating part for those with mental health concerns is that almost all the current medications available have their own unique, often unpleasant side effects, leaving them discouraged with the conventional methods of treatment available. They must choose which is worse, their symptoms or the side effects of their medications. As such, many have begun to explore alternative treatments, which includes plant medicine.

Now, after almost seventy years, we are back where it all began. Back to the sacred medicines that have been used for centuries in ceremonial settings and, more recently, explored during the early years of modern psychiatry. Yet we are still asking questions such as: What do psychedelics actually do within the body? What roles do psychedelics have in our minds and moods? How can we best utilize these changes to improve our lives? Who should have access to such powerful substances? In what ways may we be able to best utilize these substances? Throughout *The Microdosing Guidebook,* I hope to answer some of these questions and explain how microdosing may be a viable option for you to take an active role in your own mental health journey.

CHAPTER 3

THE BIOPSYCHOSOCIAL MODEL OF HEALTH

BIOLOGY
Physical needs
Genetics
Drug effects
Diet

PSYCHOLOGICAL
Mental health
Self-esteem
Coping skills
Distress tolerance

SOCIAL
Social circles
Work relationships
Family
Community

Just as people are a microcosm of something bigger than themselves, we now have come to the realization that optimal health is dependent on various other factors than one's physical health. This was not always the case. Once upon a time medical professionals thought that all physical ailments were due solely to a physical/biological reason or pathology; this was known as the biomedical approach to medicine. It wasn't until the late 1970s that medical professionals began to understand how people are more than their physical entity, and their healthcare is influenced by more than just medical applications (i.e., medications, surgery, exercise, diet, and mental well-being).

The biomedical approach to medicine was all well and good until you started to consider how all living things that have love, care, support, and a sense of connection to others often had better health outcomes than those without these advantages. This phenomenon is not unique to humans. It has been seen in plants and animals alike. Studies have shown that monkeys who were isolated from others exhibited depressive symptoms and isolative behaviors. Why would humans be any different? Are you familiar with Maslow's "hierarchy of needs"? A sense of belonging and love is in there for a reason.

Then, in 1977, we saw the development of a new approach to healthcare, what is now known as the biopsychosocial model, which looks at the whole person. This includes the person's environment, how they fit within their environment, and their social interactions with others. With this holistic approach to healthcare, individuals ultimately have better health outcomes, both physically and psychiatrically, compared to treatments that only address one's physical concerns. These improvements have been explored for various health conditions including the management of pain, depression, cardiac health, and various other medical conditions. The differences show statistically significant improvements when using a holistic approach compared to treating the condition alone.

The biopsychosocial model further describes that if an individual experiences a deficiency in one of the three realms (biological, psychological, or social), the components of the other two realms may be affected as well. Thus, the individual may experience poorer outcomes overall. Conversely, by improving or enriching one of the three realms, the other areas may also show improvement, thus resulting in overall better outcomes. One thing to note, many may include a fourth component, the spiritual component, which includes an individual's soul as well.

I won't get too in depth in regard to the spiritual realm of this model, but some have reported significant shifts in their spiritual well-being and beliefs as a result of psychedelic use. This is often after high doses or macrodoses of psychedelics, in which mystical experiences are induced, but there are some reports of this occurring with microdosing psychedelic medicines as well. This is often associated with increased connectivity or the sense of oneness with others.

Given my background and experience in holistic nursing modalities, it is the biopsychosocial approach and mindset that *The Microdosing Guidebook* program takes. I see and use this approach every day and have observed drastic improvements in many as a result. This is what I feel is exciting about this guidebook—not only are you going to gain the information on how to microdose safely, but you are also going to learn ways to look at life differently and harness the power these sacred and magical substances impart, which may help you enact lifelong changes.

SELF-CARE

One significant and often overlooked way to improve one's overall health is by performing self-care. Self-care can be anything such as exercise, reading, talking with a friend, sitting on the beach, or meditation. The important part is you are taking time for yourself.

Self-care is what people do for themselves to establish and maintain health, and to prevent and deal with illness. It is a broad concept encompassing hygiene (general and personal), nutrition (type and quality of food eaten), lifestyle (sporting activities, leisure etc.), environmental factors (living conditions, social habits, etc.), socio-economic factors (income level, cultural beliefs, etc.) and self-medication.
—The World Health Organization, 1998

One of the biggest misconceptions is that self-care is a selfish act. Self-care is not selfish; it is necessary to prevent burnout and fatigue. This concept is difficult for many to comprehend, especially when talking about themselves.

One way to visualize self-care is to think of yourself as a glass of water. As you pour a little bit of that water into everything, you give from yourself (e.g., to family, work, school, life in general). Eventually, the cup starts to run dry and there will be nothing else to pour out. Self-care activities are the things in our lives that enable us to refill that cup, thereby making us sustainable and resilient. In that sense, denying yourself the ability to perform self-care activities is actually doing yourself a disservice in the long run. Self-care can also lead us to be more present in the moment for those around us.

In the workbook section at the end of this book, there is space to brainstorm ideas for your own self-care and strategies to incorporate them into your everyday life.

THE FOUR PILLARS (AKA FOUR FOOD GROUPS) OF MENTAL HEALTH

Like houses, people need to have a strong foundation to build upon in order to remain stable and resilient in the face of storms, chaos, and the everyday struggles of life in general. I believe that one of the best ways to build stability is through establishing a consistent routine, which can minimize disorder.

Another element that I feel is extremely important for maximizing outcomes is what I like to call the Four Pillars of Mental Health (aka Four Food Groups of Mental Health). Individually, these four components are solid bases to build upon, but as you will see, they are still interconnected. These four components are diet, exercise, sleep, and stress/anxiety management.

DIET

Diet is referred to as the food or drink that one takes into their body. But if you take it from its Latin and later Greek origins, diet comes from *diaita,* which translates into "a way of life." In this sense we can understand how diet means more than just what is taken by mouth and technically is anything taken into the body. This would include not only food or drink but also how one takes in sensory information, be that from books, TV, social media, bright lights, smells, and sounds. Anything taken in from the sensory organs can be included as part of one's diet.

We have begun to understand how other stimuli such as screen time, video games, and any other modern technologies affect us both physically and mentally. In studies, we have seen how our reward pathways (e.g., dopamine) are "lit up" from video games and gambling. We have also learned that screen time before bed (e.g., TV, computers, cell phones), via the blue light emitted, causes a reduction in melatonin production. Melatonin, a natural hormone produced in the pineal gland, helps regulate one's normal circadian rhythm (aka sleep-wake cycle). While this section is about diet, not sleep, this is just one example of how diet and sleep are interconnected.

As such, we should be mindful in making healthy choices and perform self-care activities to help restore the depletions that occur as a result of our entire diet.

EXERCISE

Without going too deeply into the physical benefits from having a healthy exercise routine, I want to briefly mention the advantages of exercise. Exercise is also important for one's mental health. Physical exertion releases endorphins from the brain. These endorphins are natural "feel-good" chemicals that bind to some of the same receptors that pain medications (e.g., morphine) bind with. Endorphins will help to naturally decrease pain sensations, improve mood, decrease stress, and improve sleep. I will discuss endorphins later on in "What Are Serotonin, Norepinephrine, and Dopamine?" on page 109.

It may seem counterintuitive, but when we feel tired or sluggish, increasing our physical activity activates the body to get up and keep moving. *This is similar to how an object at rest will stay at rest, but an object in motion will stay in motion.* Ultimately, increasing physical exertion can lead to a more restful night's sleep as well. So, get up and get that body moving.

SLEEP

Individual sleep needs vary from person to person, but the average person requires six to eight hours a night. One thing that is for certain: sleep is an absolute necessity. Deep slow-wave sleep (stages three and four of the sleep cycle) are the stages where the body is immobile and respirations become deeper and longer. It is during these stages that the body starts to heal itself, hormones are released (resulting in muscle growth and affecting our appetite), and the mind is unpacking information gathered throughout the day.

Neither drugs nor napping can account for what deep, restorative sleep does for both the mind and body. Some short-term effects of sleep deprivation include memory issues, cognitive declines, difficulty with problem-solving, and diminished stress management. Over time, sleep deprivation can lead to physical and psychiatric issues such as cardiac changes, weight gain, depressive symptoms, and even psychotic symptoms. No matter how much you try to fight sleep, one's physiological body requires it.

Some ways to help manage sleep disturbances are through practices known as "sleep hygiene." These include limiting napping during the day, maintaining routine sleep practices (including going to bed and waking up at the same time daily), physical exertion during the day, minimizing screen time (because of the blue light emitted) at least one hour before bedtime, minimizing caffeine intake before bed, minimizing alcohol intake (alcohol actually disrupts the ability to get into deep sleep states), and the use of soft, ambient sounds. There are some great free guided-meditation apps available online that could help you, too!

If you require short-term use of medications for sleep, remember they are not intended to be used for long periods of time. Non-pharmaceutical alternatives should be explored first, most importantly improving sleep hygiene practices and other techniques, such as incorporating mindfulness exercises.

STRESS/ANXIETY MANAGEMENT

Short-term, intermittent stress and anxiety can be helpful for drive, motivation, and activating our "fight or flight" response. But over time, chronic elevated stress can result in increased levels of cortisol (a hormone that can lead to weight gain and hinder muscle growth), changes in mental health, and cause long-term health issues such as elevated blood pressure, ulcers, and cardiac problems.

Improving stress resilience can minimize the impact that stress has on one's overall well-being. Stress resilience helps decrease stress from building up and negatively impacting our overall health. While self-care is associated with all four of the pillars of health, practicing self-care activities is arguably the most impactful for decreasing stress and anxiety. Engaging in self-care activities help to improve one's overall health and one's ability to remain in the moment.

Stress and anxiety management also encompasses socialization and interaction. Humans are social creatures by nature. We require interaction and a sense of connection with others. Prominent mycologist Paul Stamets proposed all living things are interconnected by a network of mycelium, sharing information, energy, and life. While humans would be part of this network connecting all living things, we also need that sense of connection with others.

CHAPTER 4

THE MICRODOSING GUIDEBOOK'S RECOMMENDED PROTOCOL

Where to start? It is my hope that through this guidebook you can find information on how best to microdose psychedelic medicines for your individual needs. Unlike the conventional medical model, microdosing can be tailored to you. During your time following the proposed protocol, it is my hope that you not only feel a benefit from microdosing, but you also build a relationship with your substance of choice. Ideally, you will begin to understand how the medicine affects you, and then you will be able to find out how much and how often you may want to dose.

IS MICRODOSING RIGHT FOR EVERYONE?

The short answer is no, microdosing is not right for everyone, but the actual safety profile of psilocybin suggests that it may be relatively safe for most individuals. Psychedelic mushrooms have been consumed safely by innumerable individuals all over the world for thousands of years. Throughout the years of research conducted with classic psychedelics (i.e., psilocybin, LSD, and mescaline), there has been no evidence showing long-term neurotoxic effects resulting from their use. When psilocybin was designated by the FDA with breakthrough-therapy status for treatment-resistant major depression, the US federal government felt that these substances were so safe that the FDA did not feel it was necessary to conduct preliminary safety studies on animals before clinical trials in humans.

While many of the classic psychedelics have been shown to be generally safe, there are still some questions and concerns that have not been fully addressed due to gaps in research. Some of these concerns are related to the effects these substances have on individuals with preexisting physical conditions such as hypertension or psychiatric conditions such as psychotic disorders or bipolar disorder. Much of the modern research has excluded individuals with these conditions due to their suspected risk of long-term effects. Specific conditions that should be considered before microdosing are described in Chapter 11 and specific considerations for your healthcare provider to consider are explored in Chapters 13 and 14.

To begin, I would like to start with the most researched and explored protocol: the Fadiman Protocol.

INTRODUCTION TO THE FADIMAN PROTOCOL

In 2011, Dr. James Fadiman, a pioneer in the field of psychedelics, published *The Psychedelic Explorer's Guide,* a how-to handbook for those wanting to learn more about psychedelic substances. Within that book, one chapter vaguely described microdosing psychedelic substances, spurring many readers to contact Dr. Fadiman directly, asking him how they, too, could microdose for their own benefit. To be clear, I am not insinuating that Fadiman came up with the idea of microdosing—in fact he attributes that to Albert Hofmann—but Fadiman's name has become synonymous with microdosing psychedelics.

In the years following the release of *The Psychedelic Explorer's Guide,* Dr. Fadiman found a renewed interest in psychedelic medicines, with a focus on microdosing psychedelics and the challenges that come with researching illegal substances. Fadiman encountered difficulty obtaining approval for his research, finding enough participants for his research, and funding the cost of conducting his work. As a result, he became creative and began working on the largest open-label, nonclinical microdosing study to date. This study has been used in nearly sixty countries worldwide and includes thousands of respondents.

THE FADIMAN PROTOCOL

The goal of microdosing is to ingest subperceptual doses of psychedelics in order to have maximum results, whatever your intention may be (for instance, to treat depression or enhance creativity) without the full-blown psychedelic trip. Currently, there isn't an accepted consensus of what is considered a microdose, but most accepted responses suggest it to be between one-twentieth to one-tenth of a normal psychedelic-inducing amount of psychedelics. Given the wide range that this dosage may be, following the proposed protocol, I will help you to find your optimal microdosing amount. For best results, I encourage you to start low, and go slow.

DOSING: Since the goal is to take between one-twentieth to one-tenth of a normal psychedelic-invoking dose, we need to establish exactly how much that is. Now, don't worry if your drug math is a little rusty, I will help break it down for you.

	FULL-TRIP DOSAGE	MICRODOSE
Psilocybin (dried)	2.4 to 3.5* grams (3.5 grams =1/8th ounce)	0.1 to 0.4 grams
LSD	100 to 250 mcg (µg)	10 to 25 mcg (µg) Fadiman: 7 to 13µg

*Note: 1 gram = 1,000 mg

Early research has shown that approximately 100 mg (0.1 gram) of psilocybin is equivalent to 1 mcg (µg) of LSD.

I would like to take a moment to stress that unless you personally manufactured your LSD, the dosages out there can vary wildly and are dependent on where you live. Additionally, dosages can vary widely from batch to batch. While one square/blotter of LSD is often thought to be 100 mcg, the dosage may be on the low end at 30 to 75 mcg or on the high end of 75 to 150 mcg, according to Bryce Koch (2021), harm-reduction nurse and director of Project Safe Audience out of Winnipeg, Manitoba.

HOW MUCH SHOULD I TAKE? While I do recommend, as mentioned, that you start low and go slow, I want to remind you that your individual response depends on numerous variables. One of the main factors to consider is that the metabolism of psilocybin is dependent on one's body weight. As such, a 100 lb. female may need a dose at the lower end of the spectrum (0.1–0.2 grams), whereas a 250 lb. man might require a higher dose (0.2–0.3 grams). In addition, one's optimal dosage may also depend on individual goals or needs. Individuals who are microdosing for their depression may want a dosage that is at the higher range to have a more stimulating effect, whereas individuals who want to increase their creativity or reach a "flow state" may want a lower dose that is less stimulating.

When microdosing, you want to take a dose that is low enough that you do not feel, or at least barely feel, like you took something—remember microdosing is dosage that is subthreshold and subperceptual. If you feel an uncomfortable body high or too mentally altered to function, then you took too much. You want to be in a "sweet spot" where you may feel improvements in your mood, concentration, or increased mental acuity, but without it negatively affecting how you function in your normal, everyday life. You should feel the effects within forty-five minutes of ingestion on an empty stomach.

Finding your personal sweet spot may take a few cycles of trial and error, but journaling can help this process. If you took too little this time, then next time try bumping up the dosage slightly. If you feel nauseous or overstimulated, next time you may want to take the dosage down a bit. I will discuss techniques that can help mitigate physical side effects with more detail as we move through this guidebook.

WHEN SHOULD I TAKE MY DOSE? Once again, everyone is affected differently, and what may be good for one person may be different for another. That being said, I recommend you take your microdose in the morning, to start. Psychedelics such as psilocybin do influence the cardiac system by changing pulse and blood pressure, which can result in a mildly stimulating response. If you dose too late in the day, you may experience sleep disturbances. Meanwhile, there are others who do not experience their microdose as being stimulating and may even begin to feel tired as a result of their dosing. These individuals may want to take their dosage at bedtime. This phenomenon is not unique to microdosing. Some report experiencing similar effects from antidepressant medications; those people have found this dosing strategy effective.

The absorption of psilocybin in the stomach depends on whether you are taking it on an empty stomach or with food. Like anything, consistency is key. Taking it similarly for a few cycles may help you to understand how it affects you physically. If you normally dose after eating breakfast without issue but then skip breakfast on a dosing day, your experience for that day may be different. For example, some people experience nausea with psilocybin and take it with food (other strategies to augment side effects are discussed later). Alternatively, if you normally microdose with food but then do not, it may hit your system quicker and result in a more stimulating effect. Understanding these effects can help foster the relationship you are trying to build with your medicine.

Two of the easiest things you can do to zero in on your microdosing needs are to establish a routine, especially on your dosing days, and to journal during the initial few weeks to understand the effects of the medicine. Journaling will help you to keep track of various factors that may be relevant to microdosing. The workbook section will help you with that.

It may also be a good idea to take your first microdose on a day you do not have to work or have too many responsibilities. You want to be able to be safe, feel comfortable, and focus on how the microdose affects you. Take note of how you felt both before and after, what you ate before, and other things that may help you to understand how the microdose is affecting you physically. Take notes throughout your day to keep a personal inventory about your body and mind. The more you understand about how the microdose affects you early on, the better you'll understand your personal dosing needs in later cycles.

DO I NEED TO TAKE THE MICRODOSE DAILY? No. Unlike conventional medications that you need to take daily (or numerous times per day) in order to be effective, microdosing psychedelics daily is contraindicated. Psychedelic substances have been shown to be unique in that the long-term changes are seen long after the substance has been removed from the body. No other medications have an action like this. In addition, daily dosing may be contraindicated due to the potential for building a tolerance to the substances. This is why many dosing protocols, including the Fadiman Protocol and the Stamets Stack protocol (page 99) recommend days when you skip taking the substances.

FADIMAN DOSING PROTOCOL

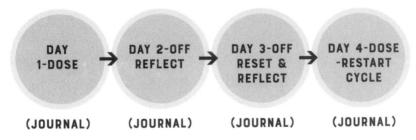

SO I TAKE MY MICRODOSE EVERY FOURTH DAY? I know it sounds odd when you may be accustomed to taking medications daily, but as shown in the illustration (Fadiman 2011, 2016, and 2018; Fadiman and Korb 2019b) and for the reasons discussed above, microdosing every day is not recommended (and may be countertherapeutic). Remember, psychedelic medicines are completely different from all other medications. So, yes, you should dose every fourth day to start.

Over time, you may find that your personal requirement is different from microdosing every fourth day, but as you build a relationship with the medicine, your body, and your unique needs, you should be able to understand what is best for you and your overall wellness.

WHAT DO I DO ON MY DAYS OFF WHEN I'M NOT MICRO-DOSING? During your "off" days, you want to take this time to reflect on how you feel without the microdose in your system. On the day following the microdose day, ask yourself: "Do I feel different?" How so?" Many report feeling an "afterglow" period after psychedelic use; this is no different when discussing microdosing. It is for this reason you want to journal. Are you experiencing an afterglow effect? Do you feel anything different at all? Do you have a couple of dosing cycles under your belt? If so, how do these reflection days compare?

On day three, two days since your last dose, ask yourself if you notice anything. That is the day you may feel like you are starting to "return to normal," and the effects of the microdose may have started to recede. It is day three that helps to reset your system and when you understand what it feels like not to have any microdosed substances in your body. Microdosing can affect some individuals for up to forty-eight hours after dosing. This pause allows your body (and neuroreceptors) time to readjust to baseline. Don't worry, day three may be more difficult, but it is only temporary. Tomorrow you start the cycle all over and microdose again.

Take this time to really notice the different feelings, understand your body, and remind yourself why you are doing this in the first place. Not every day can be a sunny day, and you can look forward to your next microdose tomorrow. But some report they still feel improved mood, creativity, and flow of energy, even on those days between dosing.

HOW LONG DO I NEED TO MICRODOSE FOR? Many report that they will continue the four-day cycle for ten cycles. At the completion of these ten cycles, you should have built a relationship with your microdose and know what your individual needs are. Many choose to continue microdosing less often and when they feel they may benefit from it (e.g., once a week or even less!).

HOW TO FIND YOUR OPTIMAL DOSE

WHAT IS THE IDEAL EFFECT? Best described by Fadiman and Korb (Winkelman 2019, 323), the ideal effect "is when you feel good, you're working effectively, and you've forgotten that you've taken anything." Like any other medication, the goal we are looking to achieve is to be effective and be able to tolerate its effects.

WHAT IF I TOOK TOO LITTLE? If you feel like you may not have hit that sweet spot in your dose, that is fine. Take this information and learn from it. In the next dosing cycle, slowly titrate the amount higher. Remember, the goal is to take subperceptual doses but still feel a benefit. This is why journaling is the key to optimal results.

WHAT IF I TOOK TOO MUCH? If you feel like you dosed too high, then during the next dosing cycle, decrease your dosage and try again. Some of the unintended side effects may include body tingling/sensations, hyperactivity, anxiety, paranoia, sweating, and loss of appetite. Decreasing the dosage may decrease these obnoxious sensations, and there are ways that you may be able to mitigate some of these unwanted side effects without lowering your dosage. These strategies are explored later in Chapter 7, "Common Side Effects and Ways to Manage Them."

If you take your microdose and then spend your day seeing dragons or can taste music, you definitely did not take a microdose. Stay calm, slay the dragon, save the princess (or prince), remain safe, and ride out the rest of the day. Enjoy the unexpected and unintended journey. If you need support for yourself or someone else, you can call:

Fireside Project: 623-473-7433 or 62-FIRESIDE

Fireside Project is a national nonprofit based out of San Francisco, founded in 2020. It is a 24/7 support hotline for people who may be struggling through a difficult psychedelic experience, supporting/holding space for others having a difficult experience, or processing and integrating past psychedelic experiences.

Additionally, next time you will definitely want to decrease your dosage… and consider purchasing a new scale.

One thing to consider: If you change the strains or the batch of your microdosing substances (e.g., mushrooms or LSD), you may need to adjust the amount you are using to microdose. The amounts of psilocybin contained within the mushroom can vary depending on the different strains of mushroom and from batch to batch. This can significantly alter the amount needed for the desired effect.

If you change your LSD supply, it would be recommended for you to reevaluate your individual dosage due to variations in consistency. Remember, LSD is not a naturally occurring chemical, nor is it legal. It is often not produced with strict laboratory guidelines and oversight; as such, there can be significant variations. Again, one square of LSD may contain on the low end 30–75 mcg of LSD, or the higher end at 75–150 mcg. This could result in accidentally taking a perceptual (or fully psychedelic) dose when actually intending on taking a microdose.

I will discuss side effects, preparation, and strains individually and more thoroughly later on.

Remember: Your individual dose may also depend on your intended goals of microdosing and what you have planned for the day. If you intend to get more work done and to concentrate, you may want to take a smaller microdose, whereas if you are hoping to get your creative juices flowing, spending time in nature (e.g., going for a hike), going to a show, or hoping to be more social or outgoing (or for some, being more introspective), you may want to take a microdose at the higher end of the range.

Taking the time to build a relationship with the medicine and to learn your individual dosage needs can allow you the freedom to make that call depending on what you feel you and your mind, body, and spirit need! This is what makes microdosing so different from other medicines, and having consistency in your microdoses (e.g., the same strain or batch) allows you to do this with freedom.

CHAPTER 5

WHEN TO START JOURNALING

While not absolutely necessary, I encourage you to journal during this time working on *The Microdosing Guidebook* program. Journaling can help you track your progress and may help you to understand more about your personal journey. As you move through this program, you will be able to look back and see how the protocol may be helping you to reach your personal goals. Like everything else in this handbook, journaling should be relevant and tailored to you (and your individual needs). I have provided blank space starting on page 183 at the end of this workbook to journal your thoughts.

I encourage you to take notes throughout the day when you begin your microdosing journey and to continue to do so briefly on your non-dosing days. If you need some ideas, try to observe your mood, mental state, any anxiety that you may be experiencing, feelings and desires, and your thoughts and perceptions. Take a moment of deep introspection into how you feel you might have changed, especially concerning those aspects you intend to change during the course of microdosing. I have included an outline for a minimalist's approach to journaling for those who may be averse to the concept; these can take less than a minute to complete.

Journaling offers you the unique ability to look back retrospectively after a few dosing cycles and see how the microdosing may have affected you, and how you may be able to make changes to your doses in order to achieve optimal outcomes. Remember, this is a long journey like hiking the Appalachian Trail, not running a 5K.

I feel journaling is even more important during times of transformation and transition to help an individual reflect on how they feel they are doing physically, emotionally, and spiritually. Take time to sit and reflect before you answer the following suggested questions, being mindful and present with your thoughts, feelings, and emotions. Here are some ideas you may wish to include to get the ball rolling.

WHAT WAS YOUR INTENTION?

How are you feeling about your journey going into *The Microdosing Guidebook* and is it affecting your set intentions? If you don't have an intention clearly in mind, don't worry. It may come in time.

MENTAL HEALTH/MOOD/EMOTIONS

How is your mood on a scale of 1–10? Do you notice that you are feeling happier? Less depressed? Do you feel like a weight has been lifted from you? Is your mood more even-keeled or does it fluctuate throughout the day? Are you able to keep your emotions in check?

SENSES

Does the world look brighter? Are you seeing better? Are you hearing better? Is your sense of smell sharper? Do things feel softer? Warmer? Do things taste better?

CONCENTRATION

Do you feel like your concentration has improved? Can you focus more easily? Do you feel like you can be more engaged in projects or tasks? Are you able to remain present in the task at hand?

ANXIETY

Do you feel more or less anxious than usual? Do you feel calmer overall? Do you feel more guarded? More fearful? On edge? Describe your anxiety; what does it feel like physically, mentally, or emotionally?

SOCIAL

Do you feel more outgoing? Do you feel like you want to be around other people more? Do you want to interact with others more than usual? Do you feel more oneness or more connected with others? Do you feel more empathetic to others around you?

INTROSPECTION

Do you feel more introspective or aware of your thoughts, feelings, actions, or the words you use? Are you more aware of your actions and how they affect your life or the lives of those around you? Are you more withdrawn personally or socially?

CREATIVITY

Do you feel more creative? Do you feel like you understand how things work better? Do you feel like you are better at seeing alternative views or approaching challenges in a different way? Have you been creating more art or writing differently? Do you feel unrestrained by mental blocks that you may have set up for yourself?

PHYSICAL

Are you exercising more? Do you feel like you have more energy? Are you sleeping better? Are you dreaming more vividly? Are you eating better? Do you drink, smoke, or take non-pharmaceutical drugs less often? Are you experiencing less physical pain?

OVERALL OUTLOOK

Overall, how do you feel things are going? Do you feel better or see things in a different light? Do you feel like you are benefiting from this guidebook? If so, how? If not, what do you feel is the issue?

EVALUATION

What should you do next? Should you continue? Was the dose too much? Or too little? Should you alter the dose for the next cycle? Should you alter the situations surrounding your dose regimen? Are you experiencing side effects? Can you make changes to mitigate those side effects?

Now that you have taken the time to reflect and journal those things, what do you do with it? I do not recommend that you make major changes in your microdosing cycle too quickly– remember this is a process. Keep these ideas in mind and you can build on them throughout The Microdosing Guidebook. *When you are ready, you will know.*

MEASURABLE SCALES

In addition to the six-week microdosing program in the workbook section, I have included a list of popular scales used within the mental health field to track improvements or perceived changes. One of the most beneficial may be the mood chart. This chart can be used to log your dosing days quickly and efficiently and to keep track of the amount microdosed, mood, your resulting experiences/side effects, and thoughts/plan.

Remember: these charts are not intended to diagnose or treat a medical condition, just to help track your progress.

Additionally, I have included the PHQ-8 for depression (Kroenke, Spitzer, and Williams 2001) and GAD-7 for generalized anxiety (Spitzer, Kroenke, and Lowe 2006). These are the standard scales that mental health clinicians use to track progress when prescribing medications for these conditions. If interested, try to fill out what you may find relevant in the personal notes section of the workbook section. Start early and try to follow up every couple of weeks to see where you have made progress. If there is something else you want to track, you can make your own list in your personal journal.

CHAPTER 6

MICRODOSING FOR PHYSICAL AND MENTAL HEALTH

As described earlier, there are three broad reasons for why an individual may be interested in microdosing psychedelic substances: to improve performance, treat a pathological condition, and decrease drug or medication use, but you may be asking yourself what some specific examples are. Contained within this chapter are some medical and psychological conditions that microdosing might treat, and ways that microdosing might improve your life.

MENTAL HEALTH APPLICATIONS

Many mental health conditions have common themes and overlapping symptoms, regardless of the actual diagnosis. One of the most common themes concerns rigid or patterned thinking.

Microdosing is often used to help with mental health conditions such as anxiety, post-traumatic stress disorder, depression, and mood swings. Microdosers say it can also be effective with ADHD, OCD, and other mental health concerns as well. Let's take a broad look at some of these.

DEPRESSION, ANXIETY, PTSD, AND MOOD

As referenced earlier, the concept of microdosing psychedelics, specifically LSD as an antidepressant, may be the earliest and best-known application. While there haven't been any conclusive long-term studies specifically looking at the use of microdosing psychedelics for the alleviation of depression, there have been more than a few studies that have reported improvements in mood by participants who have microdosed. This may be due to breaking an individual's rigid or concrete thought patterns and changing the way they see the world around them. Later, in "Psychotherapy and Microdosing" on page 82, we will come back to this theme and why changing these rigid patterns of thought are necessary to make long-term shifts, and how these effects are different from standard treatments such as conventional antidepressant medications.

Since these mental health symptoms are some of the most popular reasons people seek out microdosing as an alternative treatment option, this guidebook will explore this area more in depth in future chapters.

ATTENTION DEFICIT, HYPERACTIVITY DISORDER (ADHD)

Some have described experiencing a sense of decreased distractibility and increased focus as a result of microdosing psychedelics. In some of the self-reported studies, participants who disclosed having been diagnosed with ADHD described experiencing improved focus as well.

James Fadiman asserted that in conversations with Albert Hofmann, Hofmann felt that had pharmaceutical companies wanted to invest time into researching microdosing, it might be as popular as methylphenidate or amphetamine salts (many may know these by one of their brand names—Ritalin and Adderall, respectively) for the treatment of ADHD. In addition, microdosing may help individuals to achieve a "flow state" or what is referred to as "hyperfocus" for individuals with ADHD. A flow state is a mental state in which a person experiences an excited focus and sense of being fully involved in the task at hand. This flow is a period of complete absorption in an activity, which also results in a loss of sense in time and space. If you have ADHD, you probably know what this state is, but microdosing may help others accomplish this state.

Currently, there is no published research directly measuring microdosing as a treatment for ADHD, but there are private companies that are in phase II clinical trials investigating microdoses of LSD for ADHD. The effects are similar to the manner that psychostimulants help those with ADHD.

OBSESSIVE-COMPULSIVE DISORDER (OCD)

Obsessive-compulsive disorder is a mental health condition that is associated with repetitive thoughts, actions, and rigid, patternistic thinking. These urges and patterns are often driven by an anxiety component; performing these tasks often helps to alleviate some level of anxiety. Conventional treatments for OCD often include antidepressant medications with concurrent psychotherapy, with the goal to break these rigid patterns of thinking. Since stimulating the 5-HT2A receptors results in a reduction of rigid patterns of thought and improvements in one's ability to adapt to change, and classic psychedelics bind to these receptors, it seems plausible that individuals with OCD may benefit from microdosing psychedelics. Initial research supports these claims as well in both mice and human studies.

It is suspected that the administration of psychedelics may cause a "rebalance" of the 5-HT1A and 5-HT2A receptors, leading to a reduction in symptoms, but this theory has yet to be proven. Currently, there is only one study that directly looked at a reduction of OCD symptoms and microdosing, but crossover symptoms should not be ruled out (see "Depression, Anxiety, PTSD, and Mood" on page 63).

SUBSTANCE-USE DISORDERS

Throughout psychedelic literature, there has been resounding interest in the use of psychedelics for the treatment of various substance-use disorders. Unfortunately, much of the research is often correlated with macrodoses and not microdoses. Psychedelics were explored as a treatment option for alcohol-use disorder and opiate-use disorders, and were almost included as a step in the Twelve-Step Program for Alcoholics Anonymous. More recently, Johns Hopkins Center for Psychedelic and Consciousness Research has been exploring the use of psilocybin for nicotine dependence and alcohol-use disorder, but more applications are expected in the near future.

Mental health and substance-use disorders have a significant number of co-occurring or overlapping presentations, symptoms, and treatment options. Sometimes from a clinical and treatment perspective, it is difficult to understand which came first and if individuals are attempting to self-medicate their mental health symptoms (i.e., depression, anxiety, sleep disturbances, etc.) through substance use. It would seem reasonable that if microdosing may be beneficial for individuals with mental health symptoms (see earlier indications described), then microdosing may also be beneficial for those battling substance-use disorders, especially if they are self-medicating.

It should be noted, research has shown that ingestion of psychedelic substances has not been linked to increased substance use. It is believed that this may be because psychedelics do not produce any significant actions on the dopamine receptors, which are responsible for the positive reinforcement piece of substance-use disorders.

INCREASED SOCIAL RELATEDNESS/ SOCIABILITY AND CONNECTEDNESS

Feelings of isolation, low self-esteem, and a sense of disconnection from others are common themes throughout many mental health disorders, substance-use disorders, and developmental disorders (including autism spectrum disorders). Arguably, improvements in these sensations may contribute to overall improvements in anyone's life and well-being.

Have you ever read or listened to Gabor Maté discuss his thoughts and theories regarding mental illness and addiction? In his TEDxTalk entitled "The Power of Addiction and the

Addiction of Power," he explains how he heavily attributes these disorders to loss, trauma, and the resulting psychological pain. Now, you may be asking yourself why loss, trauma, and psychological pain are included in a section about social relatedness and connectedness? It is because of Gabor Maté's (TedxTalk 2012) declaration that "the opposite of addiction is not sobriety, but connection." Perhaps by improving these sensations through microdosing, we may see improvements in so many other conditions?

MEDICAL APPLICATIONS AND MICRODOSING

Although microdosing is often associated with mental health conditions, it may be beneficial for many other health concerns, some of which may be novel applications as well. Many of these applications are due to the downstream physiological effects resulting from the agonism (stimulating) serotonin 5-HT2A receptors, including stimulation of both neurogenesis (the process of forming new neurons or connections within the brain) and increases in brain-derived neurotrophic factor (BDNF) in the brain. These are explored more thoroughly in the subsequent sections.

REDUCTION IN NEUROINFLAMMATION

Neuroinflammation is an inflammatory response within the brain and/or spinal cord. It can be due to various conditions, including physical traumas (e.g., traumatic brain injury or concussions), pollution, toxic exposure, and infections; also, medical and mental health conditions such as depression and Alzheimer's have been shown to elevate markers of inflammation within the central nervous system (CNS).

Exploring the relationships between inflammation and psychedelics is not a new concept; in fact, it has been researched throughout the years. In one of the earlier studies examining this concept, researchers were able to show how LSD is able to interfere with the production of antibodies in rabbits. We are now starting to understand how the ability of psychedelic substances to specifically target the serotonin 5-HT2A receptors may elicit optimal and novel outcomes for anti-inflammatory properties. One example of this is with Alzheimer's disease, which is discussed more thoroughly in "Treatment of Neurodegenerative Diseases" on page 69.

NEURAL PLASTICITY

Initial studies have shown that serotonergic psychedelics, by way of stimulating the serotonin 5-HT2A receptors, promote functional and structural neural plasticity. Neural plasticity is the nervous system's ability to change and adapt over time. Changes in neural plasticity occur from the growth of new neurons in the brain, increasing the size and density of existing neurons, and growing new neural pathways (connections within the brain).

While it is not clearly understood what effects microdosing may have on neural plasticity, early research has shown promise in this area. In one recently published study, low-dose LSD administration has been shown to increase brain-derived neurotrophic factor (BDNF) in blood plasma levels in healthy volunteers.

BDNF is an important modulator for synaptic plasticity and the release of neurotransmitters. Changes in BDNF have been associated with various processes, including management of pain, learning, memory, stress, and cognitive functioning. In addition, changes in BDNF have been specifically correlated with mental health conditions (e.g., depression, schizophrenia, OCD) and medical conditions (e.g., Alzheimer's, multiple sclerosis, epilepsy, and aging). Much like microdosing, a lot of what is known about BDNF and its role for many of these conditions is still in the early phases of research. Finding novel approaches for pain management and these medical conditions would be amazing not only this field of science, but also for those who suffer with conditions that have limited treatment options. These applications may be the next big thing for the use of psychedelics as medicine and bring many new players into the field.

TREATMENT OF NEURODEGENERATIVE DISEASES

Neurodegenerative diseases are disorders in which portions of the central nervous system progressively and irreversibly deteriorate. Presently, there are no treatments that completely stop or reverse the damage; they only slow the progression. Some of these conditions include Parkinson's, Alzheimer's, multiple sclerosis, and amyotrophic lateral sclerosis (ALS, aka Lou Gehrig's disease).

Microdosing, compared to standard or full-dose psychedelics, may be particularly beneficial for individuals with dementia or Alzheimer's as these patients may not be able to tolerate the effects of full-dose psychedelics, either physically or psychiatrically. In fact, microdosing may also be beneficial for improvements in impulse control and overall well-being in individuals with dementia due to top-down control, meaning they may become more conscious of the decisions they make before reacting. These changes in neural networks may show improvements in mood, cognition, and behaviors. While these improvements may be beneficial for various medical and mental health conditions, they may be novel treatments for individuals with dementia and cognitive impairments, because these conditions are notoriously difficult to treat by conventional means: anxiolytics, antidepressants, or antipsychotic medications.

In addition, it has been proposed that due to the anti-inflammatory effects of psychedelics through the activation of the 5-HT2A receptors, since many of these receptors are specifically located in the brain, psychedelic substances may be uniquely suited for targeting brain tissues.

TRAUMATIC BRAIN INJURY, CHRONIC TRAUMATIC ENCEPHALOPATHY, AND CONCUSSIVE SYNDROMES

Both traumatic brain injuries (TBIs) and concussive syndromes are traumatic events that occur from some form of blow to the head. These conditions can lead to cognitive symptoms such as confusion, and may include other symptoms such as headache, coordination problems, memory loss, nausea and vomiting, dizziness, sleep disturbances such as excessive fatigue, and overstimulation of the senses (e.g., disturbances from bright lights or increased sensitivity to noises).

Chronic traumatic encephalopathy (CTE) is a term for brain degeneration that is thought to be caused by repeated blows/

traumas to the head. CTEs and their effects are not completely understood at this time, and a definitive diagnosis cannot be made until a postmortem autopsy is performed on the patient. CTEs have recently come to the forefront due to several high-profile cases that CTEs were thought to have contributed to, including former WWE pro wrestler Chris Benoit's suicide and double murder of his wife and son in 2007, former NFL player and convicted murderer Aaron Hernandez's changes at the end of his life, and various others who have reported personality changes after suffering numerous impacts to the head.

Recently, there has been increased interest in using psychedelics for the treatment of these conditions for many of the same reasons discussed in the previous sections: reduction in neural inflammations, neural plasticity, and neurodegenerative diseases.

The application of psychedelics for head traumas and TBIs has gained traction with more pro athletes discussing their use in their healing process. One of the more vocal is former NHLer turned psychedelic advocate Daniel Carcillo, who has openly praised the power of high-dose psilocybin after suffering numerous concussions throughout his career.

Despite the significant waves of excitement being reported in regard to high-dose psychedelics, there are some who have more quietly voiced interest in exploring microdoses. One of those is current president of the Ultimate Fighting Championship (UFC), Dana White. In early 2021, White announced that the UFC has actively approached the research team at Johns Hopkins University about partnering with them on microdosing research, stating: "They're micro-dosing [sic] psychedelics and they're saying that it's helping some of these guys with brain injuries," White said. "We've talked to Johns Hopkins and we're working on getting us involved with that too.... The list goes on and on of all the things that we've done to try to improve the sport" (Baer 2021).

At the time of publication, where this collaboration currently stands is not entirely clear, but with increased partnerships and private investments moving into academic research, we may see these applications going forward quickly.

AUTISM SPECTRUM DISORDER

Autism spectrum disorders are a variety of neurodevelopmental conditions that manifest as impairments in social communication and/or social interactions. Psychedelics may be beneficial for individuals with autism due to the same reasons discussed in "Increased Social Relatedness/Sociability and Connectedness," on page 66.

While the concept of utilizing psychedelic medicine by individuals with autism may seem bizarre, it is not a new concept. During the period between 1959 and 1974, when psychedelics were legal, there were several studies that explored this exact theory and rationale. There had been initial microdosing research conducted with rats, which resulted in increases in both prosocial behaviors and empathy, leading researchers at McGill University in Montreal to announce their plans to explore this idea in humans.

Microdosing researchers James Fadiman and Sophia Korb (Winkelman 2019) assert that individuals on the autism spectrum did not seem to have any benefit from microdosing; many participants revealed their intention to escalate their dosages—including dosages that would no longer be considered a microdose—to see if a higher dose produced a response. As of the publication of this guidebook, no follow-up reports have been published.

PAIN RELIEF

Pain is defined as physical sensations of suffering or discomfort. Pain is a unique sensation as it is often experienced in different ways depending on the individual. One's ability to tolerate pain varies as well. An individual's ability to tolerate pain, physical or psychological, is influenced by various factors, including personal experience, trauma, cultural background, and the presence of the body's natural pain blockers (i.e., endorphins).

Another factor to consider is that psychological pain (i.e., psychological distress, anxiety, or agitation) can manifest as physical pain, also referred to as somatic pain. As such, psychological and emotional distress should be taken into consideration when discussing pain, since they can influence pain tolerance and factor into the overall experience of pain.

Dismally, many approaches for the management of chronic pain have been found to have noxious side effects (i.e., the high potential for abuse of opioids, addiction, constipation, and their influence on the respiratory system), and sometimes, individuals who chronically require pain medications develop a tolerance to the medication, necessitating escalating dosages over time to maintain the same pain control. Eventually, an individual's pain tolerance may decrease as well, complicating effective treatment options.

Given the varying types of pain, a range of nonconventional pain-management techniques have been explored. Some of these techniques utilize alternative pharmacological actions or pain pathways for either primary or adjunctive treatments. Some examples are anticonvulsants such as gabapentin or antidepressants such as duloxetine or amitriptyline.

The thought of utilizing psychedelic substances for analgesia and pain management is not a new concept. This was explored in the early 1960s by Dr. Eric Kast, who realized that many of his end-of-life cancer patients in excruciating pain found relief from LSD therapies (Kast & Collins 1964; Kast 1966; Kast 1967). Kast recounted that not only was pain diminished in these participants, most likely due to some of the psychedelic's anti-inflammatory properties, but many participants reported they found peace and tranquility after returning from the psychedelic journey they had embarked on. These patients viewed pain differently, changing their relationship with the pain.

Excitingly, microdosing may be beneficial for individuals for the management of pain due to this unique mechanism of action at the 5-HT2A receptors. Utilizing this pathway for pain management would be novel because theoretically it is more of a two-pronged approach. The first, more conventional facet is through altering the physiological response (the anti-inflammatory effects of psychedelics). The second prong, which makes this approach novel, is through changing the individual's relationship with the pain experienced or viewing the pain differently. Changing the pain experience may be attributed to similarities in the ways psychedelics can alter rigid thought patterns.

The use of serotonergic psychedelic substances, such as psilocybin and/or LSD, would provide a unique advantage over many of the other pharmaceutical interventions for pain management because they do not activate a dopaminergic response. The activation of dopamine receptors, which occurs with many conventional pain-management techniques (e.g., opioid medications) ignites the reward system in the brain, reinforcing their addictive properties and making this treatment option less than ideal. There has been one initial study conducted by the Beckley Foundation that found promising results specifically for microdoses of LSD (20 mcg) to decrease experienced pain (Ramaekers et al. 2020).

CLUSTER HEADACHES AND MIGRAINES

Individuals with cluster headaches (described as experiencing two or more periods of daily headaches for a month or more) have been found to have longer periods of remission as a result of microdosing tryptamines—classic psychedelic substances such as psilocybin and LSD are within this medication class.

Microdosing psychedelics has been studied for these types of headaches, and many people have found great benefit from incorporating a microdosing regimen; further, there are specific dosages and recommendations to follow. I've included this information and the cited sources in the provider section of this guidebook. If you feel you may benefit from incorporating this plan, please review that with your healthcare provider and come up with a personalized plan together. Cluster headaches are discussed in more depth in the Special Considerations section on page 143.

PHANTOM LIMB PAIN

Phantom limb pain refers to painful sensations in an appendage that is no longer present on the body. The limb is gone, but the feeling of pain is real. The experienced pain often begins shortly after the limb has been removed by surgery or from a traumatic accident.

The research on psychedelics to treat phantom limb pain is limited, and the sample sizes are quite small, but this may be an area that can significantly benefit with further research.

In one small study of seven participants, five found improvements in pain and a reduction in analgesic use following treatment. Two of those five had "striking" improvements, described as not needing analgesics, and the other three had pain and analgesic use reduced "moderately"— their analgesic use was cut in half. Two participants found no relief. Participants were given low-dose LSD (between 25 and 50 mcg[3]) daily (Fanciullacci, Bene, Franchi, & Sicuteri 1977).

It is not clear what changes or actions occurred to facilitate these effects. Are the improvements due to the participants' changes in ways of thinking? Their visualization or views of the pain? Changes in inflammation response? Changes in the pain pathways? Whatever the reason, continuing to reexplore these with consistent outcomes could have major implications moving forward.

PREMENSTRUAL SYNDROME AND PREMENSTRUAL DYSPHORIC DISORDER

Premenstrual dysphoric disorder (PMDD) is similar to premenstrual syndrome (PMS), but the symptoms are more extreme. Both PMS and PMDD can have physical symptoms (e.g., muscle cramps, fatigue, bloating, and headaches) and psychological symptoms that can accompany it (e.g., depression, intense

---

3. Note, this dose is slightly above the previously defined range for a microdose.

irritability, and anxiety). The current treatment for PMDD often includes selective serotonin reuptake inhibitors (SSRI) medications—the most commonly prescribed antidepressants—to help with the psychological symptoms, and anti-inflammatory pain medications for the physical ailments). Both treatment options, singularly or together, may not be enough for all women suffering from these conditions to achieve full symptom relief. Even then, women may experience negative or unpleasant side effects resulting from these standard treatment options.

Although there is a dearth of publications regarding these indications directly, Fadiman and Korb (Winkelman 2019, 324) recount one testament they received from a woman, who wrote:

> *"I wanted you to know of something that might interest you. During the month that I was microdosing, I had my periods, which have always been painful and crampy. For the first time that I can remember, it was totally normal."*

Fadiman then wrote back to inquire more, to which she responded:

> *"I only microdosed during the single month. I have not done any since. However, my periods have remained normal. You have changed my life. Thank you."*

We need to be mindful this is just one anecdotal report, but in subsequent reports, numerous women also dealing with issues of PMS/PMDD attribute having experienced improved monthly cycles as a result of their microdosing. Microdosing may be an effective treatment for PMDD due the psychological effects from serotonin activation, and the physical symptoms may be mitigated due to the anti-inflammatory effects that result from stimulation of the 5-HT2A receptors.

ANOREXIA NERVOSA

Anorexia nervosa (AN) is a psychiatric condition that has the highest mortality rates and the highest cost for treatment of all mental health disorders. Conventional treatment options for AN are limited and found to be marginally effective. Cognitive behavioral therapy (CBT) is the most widely used treatment modality for adults, but remission rates are still over 50 percent. In addition, currently there are not any approved pharmacological treatment options for anorexia. Most pharmacological interventions target AN's accompanying symptoms (e.g., depression, anxiety, and rigid-thinking patterns), utilizing either atypical antipsychotic medications and/or antidepressant medications. These methods have been shown to have limited efficacy for increasing an individual's body mass index (BMI), stabilizing weight, or reducing accompanying symptoms (e.g., OCD, depressive symptoms, or anxiety).

Some have proposed the use of psilocybin, given the psychedelic's ability to uniquely target the accompanying symptoms (anxiety and depression) and the rigid-thinking patterns associated with anorexia. In theory, psilocybin may have the ability to normalize dysfunctional neurobiological systems, decrease the anxious and rigid avoidance of food, and in turn lead to healthy weight gain, resulting in long-term recovery. As of publication, phase I clinical trials exploring large-dose psilocybin for AN have begun.

I want to note, these proposed interventions and clinical trials regarding AN and psilocybin are for large dosages, not microdosing amounts, though like much of the microdosing literature, there is a lack of literature on this specific condition. But microdosing psychedelics may be a viable alternative worth trying for individuals with AN given their unique ability to improve mood, anxiety symptoms, and cognitive flexibility.

OTHER MEDICAL APPLICATIONS

Microdosing may help to treat other medical or health conditions because of the physiological changes that occur from the stimulation of serotonin 5-HT2A receptors. If proven successful, many will be able to access novel treatment options and become active participants in their personal healthcare regimen. In addition, microdosing has the added benefit of often costing less than many conventional medications and often offering fewer side effects.

Microdosing is not a panacea or cure-all for all ailments, but it may be many have more medical uses not covered in this guidebook. Further research into specific conditions may be beneficial and may lead to novel treatments for various conditions such as rheumatoid arthritis, asthma, fibromyalgia, post-treatment Lyme disease syndrome (formerly known as chronic Lyme disease), and other disorders associated with inflammation responses or markers of inflammation (including depression). There may be other ailments yet to be explored that are related to effects occurred from agonism of the serotonin 5-HT2A receptors, such as neurogenesis, neural plasticity, expression of BDNF, dendritic growth, etc.

We can also begin to look at exciting potential implications for mental health conditions, personality changes, and more, if microdosing is coupled with psychotherapeutic interventions. That will be coming in the "Psychotherapy and Microdosing" on page 82.

MISCELLANEOUS OTHER APPLICATIONS

We discussed specific mental health conditions in the previous section, but microdosing may improve other applications that are not strictly "clinical" conditions. Let's take a look at some of these hypothetical applications, which may benefit the "walking well"—individuals without pathological conditions. It is my opinion that microdosing psychedelics in general can help many improve their lives and should not be relegated to those with a clinical diagnosis.

PERFORMANCE ENHANCEMENT

As mentioned previously, microdosing may help individuals to achieve improved focus or flow states of thought. Microdosing may increase productivity in work, improve time management, and enhance the ability to learn new material. The application of these benefits may be unlimited and highly personal to an individual's skills or abilities.

COGNITION: CREATIVITY/CONVERGENT AND DIVERGENT THINKING

Cognition is the ability to gain knowledge, experience, and to learn. Some common themes reported by individuals who have microdosed were a sense of improved cognition and changes in their patterns of thinking. These claims have been well documented for *macrodoses* of psychedelics. One theory is that macrodoses of psychedelics improve or alter patterns of thinking, problem-solving, and how individuals approach challenges, which in turn improve mental health symptoms such as depression or substance-use disorders. Early research seems to indicate that this translates microdoses to as well.

Cognition should also be taken into consideration when discussing depression, mood, anxiety, and other mental health conditions, since these issues are correlated with cognitive slowing. Aging and medical conditions, such as Alzheimer's and Parkinson's disease, which we discussed earlier, also relate to a decline in cognition.

PERSONALITY CHANGES AND EMOTIONAL INSIGHT

Unlike conventional medicine, psychedelic medicines (in both macrodoses and microdoses) have been shown to induce significant personality changes and improved emotional insight for users. The "Big 5" personality traits (agreeableness, conscientiousness, extraversion, neuroticism, and openness) are generally considered ingrained and not expected to change easily or in a short time span. In addition, introducing microdosing into one's life may help to facilitate change and aid in one's ability to gain insight into personal issues one may need to work through.

Along with facilitating change, microdosing may also help individuals to identify, process, describe, and express their emotions more easily and with more accuracy. These skills and abilities may further improve as one learns to understand and integrate their emotions in more meaningful ways. Other changes observed from microdosing are an increased consciousness (reporting more organization, feelings of responsibility, and determination) and a diminished sense of procrastination in performing tasks. These concepts are explored in more depth later in this chapter.

PSYCHOTHERAPY AND MICRODOSING

The application of low, subperceptual doses of psychedelic medicines have long been theorized to be beneficial as a supplement to psychotherapy. But, when applied in practice, the results have been mixed. Unlike many of the other applications discussed throughout this book, the use of psychedelics as an adjunct to psychotherapy, regardless of the dosages, may be the most extensive use yet explored. We need to be mindful of the dosages used in these published accounts, however, as they may be low dose (whereby individuals feel effects), not microdoses.

Some of the earliest reports of microdosing to assist psychotherapy were conducted by German psychotherapists who gave 20 to 25 mcg of LSD to patients to take daily for a few days prior to psychotherapy sessions. In 1953, W. Frederking reported that he found those who took LSD leading into therapy progressed faster than those who did not. In addition, when Sandoz first began producing psilocybin as medication, researchers discussed using low doses as an aid for psychotherapy. Like Frederking, they encouraged low dosages daily for three days prior to beginning psychotherapy.

Little is known how effective this was exactly, but reports did show promising results.

Taking into consideration the effects of stimulating the serotonin 5-HT2A receptors by psychedelic substances (i.e., less rigid patterns of thinking, excitability, enhanced emotional processing, and disruption of normal consciousness), microdosing during times of concurrent psychotherapeutic treatment may improve clinical outcomes. If so, this may be similar to some conventional treatment options for many mental health issues—concurrent SSRIs and psychotherapeutic interventions. This concurrent treatment is encouraged because it is more successful than either method alone.

One popular theory for why microdosing and psychotherapy may be an ideal pairing is that microdoses lower the imaginary barrier between our conscious and unconscious mind, allowing information to stream with ease. Microdoses may allow access while maintaining the ability to read and write, perform mundane tasks, and focus on conversations (allowing increased exchange of ideas), and may also be beneficial for individuals who have a shorter than average attention span.

Further, psychotherapy may be necessary to maximize the improvements in neurogenesis and neuroplasticity that are afforded from microdosing. Sure, we may have the benefit of growing and strengthening neurons in the brain and making new connections, but the psychotherapeutic benefits may be in learning new ways to utilize these connections.

Concurrent microdosing and psychotherapy is one area that I hope to see explored further. Improved technology, communication between researcher groups, and improved research modalities may help us to better understand the benefits of these practices. It is my belief that anyone can benefit from the skills and knowledge gained from engaging in some form of psychotherapy. I understand that not everyone has access to these treatments, and many are not open to engaging in psychotherapy, but I encourage you to consider it, if for nothing else than to maximize your potential gained from microdosing. If you choose not to, however, engaging in some form of "contextual manipulation" or challenging your own fixed, rigid thoughts or beliefs may optimize outcomes. This is why I included the workbook portion of this guidebook—to help you learn ways to address some of the common themes in the biopsychosocial model in order to accompany your microdosing journey.

As Dr. Robin Carhart-Harris (Buller and Moore 2021), a psychologist, neuroscientist, and psychedelic researcher, said describing the integration of psychedelics and psychotherapy: "This combination treatment is fundamentally a biopsychosocial treatment."

REPORTED BENEFITS FROM MICRODOSING (BASED ON SUBSTANCE USED)

Throughout this book, I have referred to the psychedelics for microdosing (psilocybin and LSD) interchangeably. This is due to the fact that, at this time, there is minimal research on specific applications of one substance being more effective than the other. Some have reported they feel LSD is "cleaner" and better suited for self-discovery or cognitive improvements. Some make reference to LSD having a more pharmacological feeling since it is made in a lab. Meanwhile, others report they feel psilocybin is better suited for physical/athletic improvements, improvements in mental health conditions, or feeling closer to others. Some also refer to how psilocybin is natural or can be grown, not synthesized. Regardless, at this point the actual differences between substances are not known nor well understood.

There has been one study (Petranker et al. 2020) that collected improvements reported by microdosers and compared the specific substances the microdosers had used. The difference in results is not significant with the exception that participants using LSD seem to report having enhanced mental clarity and memory improvements compared to psilocybin (45% vs 29%).

REPORTED EFFECTS FROM MICRODOSING

In a smaller study (Cameron et al. 2020), participants reported changes in various areas of mental symptoms, which were either improved, worsened, unchanged, or unknown when a response was not given. Overall, participants either found improvements or their symptoms did not get worse from microdosing. We will explore these findings again in the next chapter when we compare conventional treatments to microdosing, specifically in relation to antidepressant medications.

	Total Sample (n=383) %(n)
DEPRESSION:	
Improvement	227 (72%)
No effect	74 (23%)
Worsening	15 (5%)
No Response	n=67
ANXIETY:	
Improvement	177 (57%)
No effect	95 (30%)
Worsening	41 (23%)
No Response	n=70
MEMORY:	
Improvement	122 (39%)
No effect	146 (47%)
Worsening	46 (15%)
No Response	n=69
FOCUS/ATTENTION:	
Improvement	184 (59%)
No effect	82 (26%)
Worsening	46 (15%)
No Response	n=71
SOCIABILITY:	
Improvement	209 (67%)
No effect	70 (22%)
Worsening	35 (11%)
No Response	n=69

* Chart based on information from "Psychedelic Microdosing: Prevalence and Subjective Effects" (Cameron et al., 2020).

CHAPTER 7

POTENTIAL SIDE EFFECTS

COMMON SIDE EFFECTS AND WAYS TO MANAGE THEM

Here is a quick rundown of the most frequently experienced adverse effects from microdosing psychedelics.

SLEEP DISTURBANCES OR INSOMNIA: Classic psychedelics have stimulant-like qualities, both physically and psychologically. Similar to other stimulants, until you fully understand how you will respond to your microdose, you may want to take it first thing in the morning. Journaling may help you to understand if the sleep disturbances are from the microdose or due to something else.

Other options include:

🌀 Dose earlier in the day.

🌀 Practice mindfulness activities (e.g., meditation or guided imagery) and incorporate good sleep hygiene practices prior to bedtime (e.g., avoid electronics/blue lights, limit caffeine intake later in the day, etc.).

🌀 Incorporate other holistic methods to wind down your day.

🌀 Decrease your dose on the next dosing cycle.

Some people experience the opposite effects, and microdosing causes them to become more somnolent or tired. If this is the case, you may want to consider trying to take your dose at bedtime. Some have found this approach beneficial. This is also a dosing strategy for some antidepressant medications.

NAUSEA: One common side effect reported by users of psychedelics (both in micro and macrodoses) is experiencing nausea shortly after ingestion. Nausea and GI upset, including vomiting, stomachaches, and diarrhea, are due to the activation of serotonin receptors in the GI system, and this occurs with many antidepressant medications as well.

Some common techniques to decrease nausea with psychedelics are:

Mushroom tea: Try adding your mushroom dose to hot water, steep, and drink. You can also try adding it to decaffeinated teas: honey, mint, and/or ginger. Both mint and ginger are natural substances that help alleviate nausea.

Lemon tek: Known by macrodosers and passed down among users, lemon tekking is the action of adding mushrooms to lemon juice (or any other acidic drinks such as orange juice).

How to lemon tek: Soak your microdose for twenty minutes, and then ingest. You could also take the lemon tek microdose and steep into tea if you wish.

The theory is that adding the mushroom fruit body to acidic juice will mimic the actions of the stomach, allowing easier digestion. Full-macrodose users have reported their effects to be quicker and more intense. It is not clear if this would be the case for microdosing, but it should be considered, which is why consistent dosing will help you understand your individual experience/effects.

ANXIETY/POOR FOCUS: Remember, psychedelics can have similar effects to other psychostimulants. As such, if you are experiencing poor focus and concentration, you may need to decrease your dose in your next dosing cycle. Taking other stimulating substances with your microdose (e.g., caffeine or psychostimulant medications) can contribute to a worsening of symptoms. It is not recommended to take them together. Some have reported not needing their normal caffeine/coffee intake on their microdosing days. You could also consider having microdose tea instead. Mindfulness practices and journaling may help you to identify other triggers that may contribute to these reactions.

Despite various common side effects reported from microdosing psychedelics, none have been found to be overly dangerous, mostly described as "annoying" or "unpleasant." I have included a quick overview of reported side effects in the table "Reported Side Effects" on page 91. To remain in line with my premise of comparing apples to apples, I have also included some comparative statistics from reported side effects from antidepressant medications.

If you recall, serotonin receptors are located throughout the body, not just in the brain and central nervous system. When we consider this, we can understand why stimulating these receptors may result in individuals experiencing physiological responses elsewhere in the body.

Side effects like agitation, irritability, restlessness, or headaches are thought to be caused by the known psychostimulating effects of the substance and from agonism of the 5-HT2A receptors. In the "Reported Side Effects" chart, information based on findings by Petranker et al. 2020 compared to the reported side effects from SSRI medications (Ferguson 2001) show some of the more bothersome reported effects for microdosing psilocybin and LSD. In the SSRI medication study, these effects were based on findings for various medications, including citalopram, fluoxetine, paroxetine, and sertraline when compared to placebos.

Admittedly, the Ferguson study is outdated, but it was chosen based on the fact that it was large and included numerous medications. Head-to-head medication comparison studies are limited and have declined significantly since the release of research by Dr. Irving Kirsch explored the efficacy of SSRI medications compared to placebos. This is discussed further in Chapter 10, "Mental Health and Microdosing." Some sections are left blank in the chart due to lack of published research giving comparable results. Ultimately, the biggest takeaway is that the side-effect profile is very comparable between psychedelics and prescription antidepressant medications.

REPORTED SIDE EFFECTS

	PSILOCYBIN	LSD	SSRI	PLACEBO
Restless/fatigue/ somnolence	8%	10.5%	>15%	5–10%
Mental confusion	8%	10%		
Reduced focus	8%	9%		
Increased anxiety	8%	7%	1–5%	1–5%
Stomach pain, headache, sleep disturbances, loss of appetite	10%	8%	>15%	10–15%
Ruminative thoughts	5%	5%		
Negative mood, irritability	3%	4%		
Dry mouth			>5–15%	5–10%
Tremor			5–10%	5–10%
Headache	Not included in study	Not included in study	>15%	>15%
Total number (n=):	2,822	4,769		

* Chart based on information from "Psychedelic Research and the Need for Transparency: Polishing Alice's Looking Glass" (Petranker et al., 2020) and "SSRI Antidepressant Medications: Adverse Effects and Tolerability" (Ferguson et al., 2001).

SLEEP AND MICRODOSING

Due to the stimulating quality of psychedelic substances, depending on your individual tolerance to stimulants (e.g., caffeine), taking a microdose too late in the day may interrupt your ability to initiate sleep. Therefore, I encourage you to be mindful of this effect when you are choosing your individual microdosing protocol and regimen. On the other hand, you may take your microdose and feel tired or sleepy as a result. If you experience increased somnolence after taking your microdose, you may be interested in dosing at bedtime instead of first thing in the morning. Everyone is different. This is exactly how antidepressant medications are sometimes prescribed—if it makes you too tired, take it at night. If it makes you too wired, take it in the morning.

Some have reported experiencing increased vivid dreams during sleep while microdosing, which could be perceived as a positive or a negative side effect depending on the person. This phenomenon is supported by research that has shown altering serotonin levels can affect dreaming. This is why you may experience changes in sleep patterns from microdosing and why this is commonly reported with antidepressant medications as well (selective serotonin reuptake inhibitors [SSRIs]/serotonin-norepinephrine reuptake inhibitors [SNRIs]). In addition, psychedelic research conducted in the 1960s found low-dose psychedelics can extend REM phases of sleep (Muzio et al. 1966, 313–324; Toyoda 1964).

While it would be exciting to see this research potentially expanded further, it gives us at least preliminary evidence that microdosing psychedelics may in fact have some physiological effects that we may not fully understand or have measured thus far.

COLOR BLINDNESS
AND MICRODOSING

Some individuals who have microdosed and are color-blind have reported experiencing "tracers" or trails following their visual field after looking at a bright light. Some have reported this the day of microdosing, and others have reported this in the days following. Many who have experienced this phenomenon have chosen to continue microdosing because this side effect was tolerable.

Conversely, those who are color-blind have reported feeling they have experienced improvements in their color recognition and perception, even citing "improves color blindness" after ingesting psychedelic substances (Anthony et al. 2020). These reports were generalized, and they did not differentiate between using microdoses or macrodoses of LSD or psilocybin. These changes may occur due to increased connections made in the brain and visual areas of the central nervous system.

DOSE-DEPENDENT
SIDE EFFECTS

Psychedelic research has repeatedly shown that physiological effects of drug administration are dependent on the size of the dose, but correlations between individuals' perceived effects (i.e., nausea, headache, anxiety) have not been studied using micro or macro doses of psychedelic medicines. It would seem reasonable to suspect that in line with the research showing physiological effects are dose dependent, perceived side effects may also be dose dependent. Further, it would also seem reasonable that if one is experiencing perceived side effects with a microdose of psychedelics, they may be able to extinguish bothersome effects by lowering or decreasing the dose amount. So, if you experience some of these side effects, you may want to consider decreasing your dosage in the next dosing cycle to see if these effects are still present or at least more easily tolerated. Understanding this may help you to dial into your individual sweet spot.

This sweet spot can be found most easily through consistent dosing. Dosing consistency means more than just the amount ingested. Other considerations include whether you've dosed on an empty stomach or whether you've recently eaten; whether you've consumed any type of caffeine (coffee, tea, caffeinated carbonated beverages); and whether your dosage was in whole fruit or ground or in a tea. Journaling your individual dose response may help you to understand the physiological effects (including side effects experienced) after dosing in the early phases of your protocol.

CHAPTER 8

HOW DO I PREPARE MY MICRODOSES?

CONSISTENCY IS KEY

As I've tried to emphasize, for optimal outcomes, you will want to maintain consistency (consistent dose, consistent dosing schedule, consistent dosing circumstances, etc.). If you normally take your microdose with a full stomach or after eating, and one day take your same microdose steeped in tea or a lemon tek, your effects may differ. Additionally, changing your psychedelic supply (due to differences from batch to batch as discussed earlier) can alter your experience, and you may need to find your individual dose once again. Journaling your individual results, especially early on while you try to hone in on your optimal dose or sweet spot, can help. Planning and preparation can help minimize adverse side effects and expedite this process. The best way to do this is to prepare ahead of time.

HOW TO PREPARE YOUR DOSE

Just like different strains of psilocybes (psilocybin-containing mushrooms) contain different chemical compositions, different parts of the mushroom fruit body (caps and stems) contain different amounts of chemicals (psilocybin) by weight. In order to minimize inconsistency between doses, I recommend you prepare single uniform doses. The easiest way is to grind your mushrooms into a fine powder using a coffee grinder.

Next, you can take the powder and either weigh it out each time you dose (you can buy a small jewelry scale online), or you can purchase a gelatin capsule kit (available online or at most health-food stores) to prepackage your doses into preweighed capsules. Making capsules not only gives the benefit of grab-and-go convenience, but it also makes for extremely discreet packaging, storage, and dosing on the go. Ground mushroom powder and capsules are less distinguishable than keeping a jar of dried mushrooms next to your coffeepot or bedside stand.

MAKING CAPSULES

How many and how much of the fruit bodies are needed will depend on your desired dosage. As an example, if you take 15 grams (15,000 mg) of dried mushrooms, grind it down, take the powder, and fill capsules at 0.2 grams apiece (size 4" capsules), you would end up with seventy-five capsules ready for dosing.

If one person takes one 0.2 gram capsule every fourth day, these seventy-five capsules would last them for ten months.

CHEMICAL COMPOSITION

If you really want to delve into the nitty-gritty drug math, you can get a rough estimate of the percent of the psilocybin content by weight. Different species have different amounts of psilocybin (and other chemicals discussed in Chapter 1, "What Is Psilocybin and How Might It Help Me?").

It is important to remember that if you change your strain of psilocybe mushroom, your dosage may change as the percent of psilocybin varies strain to strain. Being mindful of this, you may need to alter your dosage amount and rechallenge to find your sweet spot dosage all over. These numbers are a rough estimate, testing would need to be conducted to find out the definitive percentages.

Average psilocybin amount by species:

🌀 *P. azurescens* has 1.78% psilocybin

🌀 *P. bohemica* has 1.34% psilocybin

🌀 *P. semilanceata* has 0.98% psilocybin

🌀 Both *P. baeocystis* and *P. cyanescens* have 0.85% psilocybin

🌀 *P. tampanensis* has 0.68% psilocybin

🌀 *P. cubensis* has 0.63% psilocybin

🌀 *P. weilii* has 0.61% psilocybin

AN EXAMPLE OF DOSING

Noted above, most mushrooms contain between 0.5% to 2% psilocybin (5–20 milligrams) per gram by dried weight. But, if you are looking to get even deeper into the "drug math" and want to get a better idea of what your dosage is, we can do that, too.

First, let's say you hypothetically have some of the most common (and one of the easiest to grow) mushrooms on hand, Golden Teacher, a strain of *P. cubensis* that contains approximately 0.63% psilocybin by dried weight. This means that in 1 gram of *P. cubensis*, there are approximately 6.3 mg of psilocybin. This is not a microdose. But if you split that 1 gram into fifths (0.2 grams each), then you would be ingesting approximately 0.126 mg of psilocybin.

6.3 mg / 0.2 gram = 0.126 mg of psilocybin

This is a microdose when we consider that research has shown that the threshold dose for subjective effects is approximated at 3 to 5 mg by mouth (Hasler et al. 1997).

Don't get bogged down in these heavy and nerdy details. I added this information in case you were reading through some of the older published research that describes the amounts of psilocybin individuals were ingesting in those studies, and you wanted to compare. Honestly, in school I never thought I would need to know how to figure out dosage calculations. I guess I was wrong, and I'm sure my teachers would have never expected it for this.

SHOULD I CONSIDER ADDING OTHER SUBSTANCES TO MY MICRODOSE REGIMEN?

The short answer is maybe. Recently, renowned mycologist Paul Stamets patented a combination of mushrooms called the "Stamets Stack" in an effort to maximize benefit. The idea of stacking is to synergize chemical substances in an attempt to have even better outcomes. Research on the Stamets Stack and stacking is still lacking, but you may find benefit.

THE STAMETS STACK

The Stamets Stack includes:

🌀 1–10 mg of psilocybin

🌀 500–1000 mg of Lion's Mane—a medicinal, non-hallucinogenic mushroom that has been found to have neuroprotective qualities and promote nerve growth factors. It is considered by many as a nootropic substance (which enhances cognition and memory, and facilitates learning). Research has shown it may help to slow or prevent dementia.

🌀 100–200 mg of niacin/vitamin B3—a supplement that increases vasodilation and flushing of the skin (which some refer to as unpleasant in higher doses). It is believed these effects help to distribute psilocybin and Lion's Mane throughout the entire body. In addition, niacin is known to carry GABA (a neurotransmitter associated with anxiety and fear) across the blood-brain barrier, which may result in mental health benefits, too.

STAMETS STACK PROTOCOL: Stamets recommends a different dosing protocol than the one I have recommended, which is based on the Fadiman Protocol. Stamets's protocol recommends five days on and two days off. Some choose to follow this protocol by taking their doses during the week and taking weekends off.

Notwithstanding, I prefer the protocol I describe over Stamets's. The protocol I propose offers the advantage of allowing individuals the opportunity to learn about their microdose and its effects, thereby building a relationship between the microdosers and their medicine. This is different from the normal Western approach of taking medication and expecting results. Additionally, it may allow more time for the medication to be out of the body, decreasing potential side effects, and it may lower a chance of building a tolerance to the medication.

CBD AND MICRODOSING

CBD has been shown to have anti-inflammatory, anti-anxiety, and analgesic effects, similar to microdosing psychedelics. There isn't any clinical data showing microdosing and CBD may work synergistically; it may seem advantageous to assume that when combined, outcomes may be better than either on their own, but they theoretically cancel one another out. Some individuals who may benefit the most from concurrent use may be those who are looking for improvements related to a head injury, trauma, autoimmune diseases, inflammatory bowel diseases, or neuroinflammatory diseases (e.g., Alzheimer's/Parkinson's) since both CBD and microdoses of psychedelics have anti-inflammatory properties.

VITAMIN D AND MICRODOSING

While outside the scope of this guidebook, I want to mention that everyone should be conscious of the health benefits of vitamin D and their vitamin D levels. Most Americans are deficient in vitamin D and taking a D supplement can be an easy fix to see improvements in mood.

CHAPTER 9

THE LEGALITY OF MICRODOSING

After discussing all the risks, side effects, and drug interactions, the most common question asked in regard to microdosing's legality. Under US federal law, psychedelic substances are classified as being Schedule I controlled substances by the United States Drug Enforcement Administration (DEA). Schedule I drugs are the most restrictive class of drugs and classified as such when they are "defined as drugs with no currently accepted medical use and a high potential for abuse." But as we are learning, neither of these statements is accurate when it comes to psychedelic medicines.

In select states and municipalities, some of these substances are becoming decriminalized in efforts led by the "Decriminalize

Nature" movement and supporters of "plant medicine" movements. These changes differ depending on your location, and some places have expanded their definition to include substances that are not naturally occurring, such as LSD and MDMA. To be entirely clear, you will need to check with your local state or city municipalities. Denver, Colorado, was the first to decriminalize psilocybin in May 2019, then the cities of Oakland and Santa Cruz, California, followed suit in June 2019 and January 2020, respectively. Other cities that have moved in this direction have been Washington, DC, November 2020; Somerville, Massachusetts, January 2021; and neighboring Cambridge, Massachusetts, in February 2021.

The largest shift in support of medicalizing psychedelic substances has been in the state of Oregon, where the voters passed Oregon ballot measure 109 in November 2020. Measure 109 makes Oregon the first state to both decriminalize psilocybin and legalize it for therapeutic use. Since then, numerous individual states and municipalities are actively attempting to decriminalize many of these substances and gaining public support along the way. As we have seen with the marijuana movement, change can be slow, but it can occur, though a federal rescheduling by the DEA may seem like it will never occur.

DECRIMINALIZATION IS NOT LEGALIZATION

I cannot emphasize enough the difference between decriminalization and legalization. Even though certain states may decriminalize a drug, it currently remains illegal at the federal level. When a substance is decriminalized, often punishments for possession or cultivation may be reduced to a fine or set as the lowest priority for law enforcement within the jurisdiction. There are often limits in amounts that one can possess, referred to as "personal use" or "personal consumption." Sales of these substances are also *illegal*. Since these substances are still illegal at the federal level, one could still be at risk for penalties by federal authorities if caught with them in one's possession.

Legalization means that once-illegal substances are now legal, but there may still be age restrictions in place or possession limits. Additionally, some state or local municipalities may require licensing for retail sales or production purposes. This is often the case regarding cannabis within individual states. Cannabis is legal in numerous states across the US, but it still remains illegal at the federal level.

An interesting note regarding the legality of psilocybin-containing mushrooms specifically: while the fungal fruit or mushroom containing psilocybin is often illegal to possess, cultivate, or transport, possession of psilocybin-containing mushroom spores is completely legal to own in forty-seven states, with the caveat of *"for microscopy purposes only."* They only become illegal once they are used to grow actual mushrooms. This means you could buy spores legally online or at local merchants in most of the United States. The three states in which spores are illegal are California, Georgia, and Idaho. Ironically, in many places across the globe, psilocybin-containing mushrooms can be found growing naturally, but once you pick them, you are in possession of a controlled substance.

Since most people do not live in areas where mushrooms or psychedelic substances are legal to grow or possess, this means one could argue that the potential side effect of microdosing could be arrest, seizure, and prosecution of illegal Schedule I substances. If you choose to microdose and live outside of decriminalized municipalities, please consider this as a possibility. Hopefully, in time, this will be less of a concern across the United States.

DRUG TESTING

You may wonder whether a microdose can show up in a drug test. Psilocybin has a short half-life and will be mostly excreted within eight hours; LSD is slightly longer, but it could be detectable in urine for up to a week. The good news is that standard urine drug screens do not test for psilocybin or LSD—they mostly are looking for marijuana, stimulants such as cocaine and methamphetamines, benzodiazepines, and opiates. In order to test for psilocybin or LSD, a specific drug test would need to be run, and the window of opportunity to have it in your system is small. Additionally, the amounts that may be in one's system as a result of microdosing are likely too low to reach the threshold causing a positive result.

THE FUTURE OF MICRODOSING RESEARCH AND PRIVATIZATION OF PSYCHEDELIC MEDICINES

The future of psychedelic medicine, which includes both macrodoses and microdoses, is unknown, but various factors are pushing the advancement of psychedelic therapies. Some of these include the medicines' unique and novel ability to treat and heal individuals, in many cases with better efficacy and fewer side effects than current therapies. But there are other factors that may be more dubious. As with anything that has the potential to make money, the psychedelic marketplace has seen financially driven moves, leaving many both unhappy and scared of the consequences. In the past year, numerous companies have launched IPOs and become publicly traded, which means by definition these companies report directly to investors, and their goals are financially driven. This complicates some of the aspects of research and publication of their findings, including an implicit conflict of interest.

This also spurs races for patenting novel treatments, proprietary compounds, production methods (e.g., companies stripping out partial compounds from mushrooms), and drug delivery systems (e.g., oral dissolving psychedelics, wearable technology, and others). This is similar to the technology used by an esketamine nasal inhaler or lifesaving EpiPen or insulin pen's autoinjector technology. Conversely, private companies can invest time, money, and resources into product development and advance the psychedelics-as-medicine movement. I'm not saying all of these companies are implicitly biased or have nefarious motives, I am saying they are still companies that need to turn a profit. I encourage you to be mindful of this, and we should keep these companies accountable.

One publicly traded company, MindMed, announced that they are in the process of developing a placebo-controlled study that will evaluate the effectiveness of microdosing LSD for immune-system response, quality of life, mood, emotional regulation, sleep quality, cognitive performance, and neuroplasticity. MindMed is also currently working on medications that can stop active psychedelic trips, and they are in Phase 2a clinical trials for microdosing LSD for ADHD. Yet another company, NeonMind, has filed pending clinical trials that will explore the use of microdosing psychedelics for weight loss. With all these companies pushing to make their mark within the psychedelic marketplace, we should remember that microdosing cannot be a panacea for healthcare. We should question motives and always check the research, and more importantly than the research, check the research's sources. The perils and pitfalls of pharmaceutical research will be briefly discussed later in this book.

LARGE DOSES PRIOR TO PARTICIPATING IN MICRODOSING RESEARCH

One common theme/factor that is mentioned throughout the microdosing research is that nearly all microdosing participants have had prior experience with their psychedelic substance, often macrodoses and prior psychedelic journeys. This begs a few questions. What effect do previous psychedelic experiences have on the individual and their microdosing experience?

Would individuals who have not had prior psychedelic experiences have different outcomes? Does microdosing reignite or reconnect the pathways that macrodoses first established? If so, what are those implications? Should individuals take a macrodose a week, two weeks, a month prior to initiating a microdosing regimen? Could individuals who have taken part in large-dose therapy sessions have a significantly larger improvement in their outcomes? Would taking a large dose prior to microdosing ignite these neural pathways in more significant ways, inciting the subsequent microdosing to keep those pathways open, akin to a team clearing brush to forge a hiking trail? These questions may one day be answered, but for now we do not know.

We have seen 60 to 80 percent of participants in the longest running post-psilocybin-assisted psychotherapy report continued reductions in depression, anxiety, demoralization, hopelessness, and death anxiety even four and a half years later, in follow-up interviews. What if microdosing could be shown to continue these improvements at a higher level? Imagine those implications.

I wonder if there are measurable differences in either outcome or how physiological changes differ between those who microdose with and without prior psychedelic experiences. Are biological and psychological improvements that occur as a result of macrodose sessions effectively maintained by microdosing, and if so, how often should one microdose? Should one have a macrodose session prior to initiating a microdosing protocol to maximize their potential outcomes? I think this would be an exciting area to explore.

CHAPTER 10

MENTAL HEALTH AND MICRODOSING

WHAT ARE SEROTONIN, NOREPINEPHRINE, AND DOPAMINE?

I want to provide a quick overview about the three main neurotransmitters, classified as "monoamines," responsible for many functions in the body, and their roles. Serotonin, norepinephrine, and dopamine are all neurotransmitters that are found predominantly in the central nervous system. These neurotransmitters are responsible for carrying information across the synapses (spaces between neurons) in the brain. Serotonin is the most important neurotransmitter when discussing psychedelic medicines because it affects mood and anxiety, and is the pathway that is activated for psychedelics to take effect. Additionally, there are minimal effects on norepinephrine and dopamine systems.

SEROTONIN

Serotonin receptors are concentrated within the (CNS), but they are found throughout the entire body, especially in the gastrointestinal tract. Serotonin has been noted to affect mood, cognition, learning, sex drive, anxiety, appetite, stress response, memory, sleep, and thermoregulation. Stimulating select serotonin receptors also causes physiological effects such as nausea, diarrhea, and vasoconstriction of blood vessels, just to name a few.

There are a few different types of serotonin (5-HT) receptors, but the receptors that the classic psychedelics are found to target the most are the 5-HT2A receptors. The serotonin system's effects are noted to be diverse, but its specific responsibility is not completely understood. The serotonin system has been described as involved everywhere but responsible for nothing.

Research has shown that when serotonin levels have been artificially reduced in the brain (e.g., from restrictive diets), the resulting effects have included individuals exhibiting increased aggression and impulsivity. Stimulating the serotonin system has been shown to diminish behavioral responses to noxious stimuli, including pain and anxiety. How serotonin regulates mood is not completely understood, but we do know serotonin is *associated* with mood. We know this because we have seen irregularities in serotonin in individuals with depression, insomnia, anorexia, Parkinson's disease, Alzheimer's, and schizophrenia.

NOREPINEPHRINE

Norepinephrine is a chemical within the body that is both a neurochemical and a stress hormone. As a neurotransmitter, it affects alertness, concentration, arousal, memory, and attention, and impacts both blood pressure and heart rate. Low levels of norepinephrine have been found to correlate with depression, ADHD, and hypotension (low blood pressure).

Classic psychedelics have not been found to impact norepinephrine, except for high-dose psilocybin. For this reason, norepinephrine will not be discussed in great depth. The important takeaway is that some antidepressant medications target both serotonin and norepinephrine receptors.

DOPAMINE

Dopamine is the neurotransmitter responsible for motivation, rewards, mobility, and concentration. Substances that target dopamine receptors (and the subsequent rewards) are what cause feel-good sensations, reinforcing addictive properties. Research has shown high-dose LSD does have some effects on dopamine, but not targeting these receptors directly, thus not causing addictive effects. Psilocybin does not appear to affect the dopamine system. It is not entirely understood how much, if any effect, LSD has on dopamine receptors when taken in microdose amounts, but it is suspected to be negligible.

Overall, these three neurotransmitters do affect various components of an individual's life, and an imbalance of these neurotransmitters can result in individuals exhibiting altered moods, altered thoughts, the ability to think and perceive the world around them, and anxiety (among other things). These concepts will be explored more thoroughly throughout this chapter.

DEPRESSION AND MICRODOSING

Clinical depression is a mental health disorder that is characterized by a persistent, low, depressed mood, loss of interest, and impaired ability to perform activities of daily living (e.g., showering, eating, functioning at work/school). Depression may manifest itself with other symptoms, including sleep disturbances, changes in appetite, weight loss or weight gain, poor concentration, and thoughts of suicide. Depression is the most common mental health disorder in the world, affecting almost 10 percent of American adults, and women are about twice as likely to be affected than men.

Despite the availability of numerous treatment options for depression (medications, psychotherapy, electroconvulsive therapy [ECT], and ketamine infusions), it is estimated that complete remission from depressive symptoms is achieved by less than 30 percent of those seeking treatment. Some factors that lower one's chance of full remission of symptoms are the length of time the depression lasts, previous depressive episodes, other concurrent medical or psychiatric conditions, and lower baseline functioning (when not experiencing a depressive episode). It is for these reasons mental health professionals encourage psychotherapy in conjunction with antidepressant medications. Concurrent psychotherapy and pharmaceutical modalities have been shown time and time again to have significantly higher efficacy rates for treatment than either method alone. This concept is discussed in "Psychotherapy and Microdosing" on page 82.

Research has shown that for many, a relapse and experiencing depressive symptoms after treatment is highly likely, and that's the reason many are encouraged to continue their medication plan long after they begin to feel better. Unfortunately for many, continuing these medications means continuing to experience unpleasant and intolerable side effects, leaving them to ponder the conundrum: "What is worse, the treatment or the illness?" This leads some to explore alternative treatment options and may just be the reason you wanted to learn more about microdosing.

Most of the pharmaceutical interventions available (for instance, antidepressant medications) focus on attempting to increase monoamines (serotonin, norepincphrine, dopamine) in the brain, thereby attempting to fix the "chemical imbalance" that occurs there. This is known as the "monoamine theory" of depression. As I will discuss at various points in this guidebook, these theories are shortsighted and self-limiting in treatment options. It is my hope that in the coming years, we will have a better understanding of depression and will be able to differentiate various types and their causes. It is my opinion that while depression has many similar presentations to various other conditions such as anxiety, substance use disorders, and psychological pain or trauma, it has become a general "catch all" diagnosis.

One thing I would encourage anyone to consider: Many of these mental health conditions do share similar genetic contributions, and these genes may help to predict an increased likelihood to manifest into a disorder. But these genetic factors do not necessarily *cause* the disorder; they merely increase one's vulnerability to a mental illness. Perhaps in order to manifest, there needs to be catalyst for this change. This catalyst may be the experience of a trauma, which may be physical, psychological, emotional, or spiritual, that ignited that genetic predisposition, leading to a cascade of effects, similar to the domino effect.

All too often individuals will attribute their bundle of symptoms to this clinical mood disorder without taking into consideration the circumstances surrounding the presentation and the role their personal behaviors, lifestyle choices, or health decisions contribute to their presentation. Often these modifiable factors are overlooked, and the resulting symptoms are pathologized, resulting in either a clinical diagnosis or a label the individual can identify with.

Despite all this, in my opinion, clinical depression is probably a spectrum of conditions, all having unique causes and presentations, thereby necessitating different treatment modalities. Without differentiating the various types, their etiology, and one's personal contributions, we have to take the approach as "if all you have is a hammer, everything is a nail" and unfortunately, given the limited tools available, that nail is pharmaceuticals, more specifically antidepressant medications.

COMMONLY REPORTED SIDE EFFECTS OF ANTIDEPRESSANT MEDICATIONS

Several side effects that are often associated with antidepressant medications; these vary depending on the specific medication or medication class. Many of these side effects occur because

114

the medications affect various neurotransmitters, often serotonin. People often cite these side effects as reasons for not continuing their medications. Some will even report that the side effects experienced are worse than the symptoms of the illness they intend to treat.

Remember, many of these serotonin receptors are located outside the CNS, in the GI tract, which is why there are common themes or body systems for the side effects reported. This is the reason that microdosing psychedelics shares some specific side effects with standard treatments for depression.

Some of the most common side effects reported with anti-depressant medications include:

🌀 Headaches

🌀 Dizziness

🌀 Nausea

🌀 Restlessness/anxiety

🌀 Sleep disturbances

🌀 Diarrhea

🌀 Dry mouth

🌀 Sexual side effects

   ○ Inability to achieve orgasm

   ○ Diminished sex drive

To be clear: I am *not* anti-medication, but I do understand why people decide to discontinue taking certain drugs. If you are interested in discontinuing your current medication regimen, that is a discussion you need to have with your prescriber before you just stop cold turkey. Abruptly stopping some medications (including some antidepressant medications) can cause withdrawal symptoms or what is referred to as a discontinuation syndrome, which introduces unique challenges and risks.

Discontinuation syndromes occur as a result of stopping medications too abruptly. Some of the symptoms of discontinuation syndrome include flu-like conditions, nausea, insomnia, imbalance, sensory disturbances, hyperarousal, and "brain zaps," which can last up to two weeks after stopping antidepressant medications. Additionally, quitting medications abruptly can result in a reemergence of depressive symptoms, including suicidal thoughts and attempts. Therefore, stopping medications should be done under the supervision of medical or mental health professionals. Together you can come up with a discontinuation plan safely and with minimal risk and discomfort.

Lastly, it's not always necessary to stop your traditional medications if you want to begin taking psychedelic medications. It may be safe to take both traditional and psychedelic medications concurrently. In some cases, microdosing can be incorporated into that plan, and many have found microdosing beneficial to eventually stopping other medications. I encourage you to be transparent with your provider, sharing the information and knowledge gained within this guidebook, so you can prepare safely.

Antidepressant medications are discussed in depth in "Antidepressants and Microdosing" on page 149.

DIFFERENCES BETWEEN MICRODOSING AND ANTIDEPRESSANT MEDICATIONS

While serotonin's effects are not completely understood, some of the major theorists agree that the function of serotonin in the brain is to help moderate stress and anxiety, while also promoting patience and coping. Of the fourteen different serotonin receptors that are currently known, it is the 5-HT1A and the 5-HT2A receptors that are most significant for the purpose of this guidebook. To a lesser extent, the 5-HT2B receptors and their role are discussed separately in "Cardiac Concerns in Microdosing," on page 139.

Elevated levels of serotonin have been found to not only manage mood, but also to help reduce impulsivity and aggression. These symptoms can be present in numerous conditions, including depression, anxiety, ADHD, and substance-use disorders, just to name a few. But serotonin may also play a role in helping individuals adapt or cope with stressful situations.

The activation of serotonin 5-HT1A and 5-HT2A receptors has both been shown to be associated with decreased depressive symptoms and an increase in the overall sense of well-being, though their means for reaching these outcomes are different.

5-HT1A RECEPTORS: The 5-HT1A receptors are believed to be responsible for reducing impulsivity, aggression, and anxiety during everyday stress. It is thought that these actions occur through increasing one's sense of resilience and patience, emotional blunting, and maintaining one's ability to tolerate stress.

Antidepressant (SSRI and SNRI) medications that target the serotonin system specifically work on the 5-HT1A receptors.

Because this causes the effects mentioned just above, it results in decreased symptoms of depression and an improved overall sense of well-being. But this is why many will report a sense of emotional blunting or an inability to "feel feelings" when taking antidepressant medications. This is also why many will experience depressive symptoms once those medications are stopped. Generally, antidepressant medications do not change anything structurally or physiologically in the long term; they just affect the chemicals between the synapses of the brain.

5-HT2A RECEPTORS: Psychedelic substances attach to the serotonin 5-HT2A receptors through the action called agonism. It is through this action that macrodoses of psychedelic substances have shown reductions in rigid and concrete thinking patterns and pessimistic thoughts. Other actions that occur from agonism of the 5-HT2A receptors include enhanced plasticity in thinking, increased environmental sensitivity, and improvements in one's ability for learning and unlearning behaviors. In addition, they have been shown to improve individuals' coping strategies, adaptability, and ability for change.

Ultimately, psychedelics have been shown to change the way individuals think, not merely dampen one's mood or change their emotional response like antidepressants do. The additional benefit is that psychedelics may allow access to parts of the brain that are susceptible to changes made through psychotherapy, allowing for the unprecedented one-two approach for improving one's mental health status. See also "Psychotherapy and Microdosing" on page 82 for more information.

EFFECTS ON MOOD VIA DIFFERENT SEROTONIN PATHWAYS

ANTIDEPRESSANT MEDICATIONS: From Serotonin 1A Activation

REDUCTION IN	ENHANCEMENTS IN	RESULTS
impulsivity	resilience	depressive symptoms
aggression	patience	sense of well-being
anxiety	stress tolerance	
emotional responses		

MICRODOSING PSYCHEDELICS: From Serotonin 2A Activation

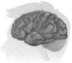

REDUCTION IN	ENHANCEMENTS IN	RESULTS
rigid thinking	plasticity in thinking	depressive symptoms
pessimistic thoughts	environmental sensitivity	sense of well-being
	learning and unlearning behaviors	
	adaptability and ability to change	
	coping skills	

Both show reductions in depressive symptoms and improved sense of well-being, but conventional treatments may dampen emotions overall versus microdosing, which actually changes the way one thinks/responds.

OTHER ADVANTAGES OF MICRODOSING VS. STANDARD ANTIDEPRESSANT THERAPIES

Microdosing may have one major advantage over standard antidepressant treatments—we may see the desired effects much quicker with microdosing due to its different actions. Some have reported seeing their depressive symptoms lift within a few days of initiating a microdosing protocol compared to the six or eight weeks that standard antidepressants often take. Also, antidepressant dosages may need to be titrated up over several weeks to find an effective dosage. During this time, many may begin to become discouraged and frustrated, and may continue to be affected by either the depressive symptoms or the obnoxious side effects of the medications. In some cases, if medications are not effective or not well tolerated, the entire process needs to start over again.

Other factors about depression and the standard methods of treatment still warrant consideration. First, many of the pharmaceutical approaches for the treatment of depression rely heavily on the chemical imbalance (or monoamine) theory of depression, and treatment is most often an attempt to increase neurochemicals (specifically serotonin) to abate the symptoms. These approaches may be ineffective if there are other causes for depressive symptoms. Second, many will get a clinical classification of having treatment-resistant depression, a term for individuals who have tried and failed two or more adequate medication trials. This term is misleading since most of the treatments tried are often similar medications (antidepressants), only targeting different neurochemicals.

The term "treatment-resistant depression" and the controversy surrounding this term have become a popular discussion point and a good reminder to both individuals living with these struggles and medical professionals. The term may be shortsighted and even disparaging, as depression can have various causes, not just a deficiency of neurochemicals, and there are actually several types of depression—those resulting from drug use or medical conditions, bipolar depression, and iatrogenic depression (side effects from prescription medications). These types of depression are unlikely to respond to conventional treatments such as antidepressant medications, and thereby may be misdiagnosed as treatment-resistant depression. We should consider whether depressive symptoms are able to respond to other forms of treatment (for instance ECT, transcranial magnetic stimulation [TMS], or vagus nerve stimulation [VNS]), and not base the term solely on failed antidepressant treatments.

In addition to all the aforementioned differences between microdoses of psychedelics and antidepressant medications, microdosing has three other distinct advantages over conventional methods of treatment. Again, these effects result from the activation of the serotonin 5-HT2A receptors, but the effects are not immediate, they have a more downstream approach and part of the cascade of changes that occur.

First, microdosing LSD has been shown to increase BDNF (brain-derived neurotrophic factor) in healthy volunteers (Hutton et al. 2020c). I specifically mention LSD because its effects have been researched in humans. Preliminary reports have found similar effects with microdosing other psychedelic substances such as psilocybin, but those other substances have been researched in rats only, though with promising results. BDNF is responsible for plastic changes related to learning and memory. These neuroplastic changes may also result in the second unique benefit: changes in the default-mode network. The default-mode network is a network within the brain that is active when individuals are not focused on the outside world—it's active during daydreaming and mind wandering, or when self-reflecting, passively watching television, or during meditation. Basically, the default mode network is active when there is no active task at hand.

Lastly, microdosing psychedelics has been shown to reduce inflammation. While inflammatory response and its role related to mental illnesses are not entirely clear, preliminary research indicates a high correlation between these conditions. More specifically, there seem to be correlations between inflammation located in the gut and gut biome, which is referred to as the gut-brain axis. This research has also indicated a reduced number of anti-inflammatory bacteria and increased numbers of pro-inflammatory bacteria within the microbiota of the gut. These relationships and the resulting effects may be the most important we may see for significant advancements in mental treatments. Microdosing's may help to reduce these inflammatory responses.

RESEARCH ON MICRODOSING'S EFFECTS

While research on microdosing's physical and psychological effects, clinical indications, and outcomes up to this point have been generally inconclusive, we do know that something is occurring, as evidenced by the measurable responses that were reported between "zero dose" and "low dose" within early psychedelic research, measurable improvements in pain response from microdosing, increased BDNF growth, and other responses described within this book.

Early in the writing process of this book, Imperial College of London announced they were attempting to conduct a self-blinding, placebo-controlled study to measure the effects of microdosing psychedelics.[4] Maybe it was serendipitous luck or

4.   Blinding means that participants do not know which substance they are ingesting, in this case they did not know if they were taking an active

maybe it was great collaboration and planning by the authors, but within mere days there were two significantly important publications discussing microdosing's effects. The first (Kaertner et al. 2021) was entitled "Positive Expectations Predict Improved Mental-Health Outcomes Linked to Psychedelic Microdosing," and then came "Self-blinding Citizen Science, to Psychedelic Microdosing" (Szigeti et al. 2021). This one-two punch was great, but I feel each did little to clear the air from microdosing's critics.

The first, "Positive Expectations Predict," basically summed up that those who had anticipated improvements from microdosing often had positive improvements, which one would expect for any treatment modality, medication or otherwise. The second, "Self-blinding Citizen Science," was a great study for researching microdosing: it had a large number of participants and attempted to blind participants. This study was stymied by the fact that an adequate study by today's standards is extremely difficult to attempt given the legal status of psychedelic medicines. Blinding was difficult and many were naturally unblinded given the fact they could identify having received active medications, a common problem throughout research, regardless of if it is psychedelic research or conventional antidepressant clinical trials.

In addition, the "Self-blinding Citizens Science" study found that nearly all participants improved due to participation of the study, whether they were receiving the active psychedelic

---

microdose or a placebo (inert/inactive substance, often a "sugar pill"). Modern standards often require a "double blind," meaning both participants and researchers do not know what participants are taking. Due to legal restraints, participants in Szigeti's team's study needed to set up a way participants blinded their own substances.

microdose or placebo, confirming the results found in the previously discussed study.

Research exploring antidepressant medications is often found to have similar issues, but these issues are not well known publicly. Due to scope of this book and to keep the focus on microdosing, I encourage you to explore some of the work by Dr. Irving Kirsch and his team (Kirsch and Sapirstein 1998; Kirsch 2008; Kirsch et al. 2008; Kirsch 2015) about the problems with antidepressant medication research and Ido Hartogsohn's (2016) work discussing the power of placebos. Some of the key takeaways from Kirsch's work compared to the microdosing research cited above include:

🌀 Kirsch and his team proved that antidepressants do in fact work to decrease depressive symptoms in many.

🌀 Kirsch and his team proved that placebos are often as effective as antidepressant medications in decreasing depressive symptoms for many.

🌀 Participants who microdosed psychedelics (and those receiving the placebo) reported improvements from mood, energy, creativity, emotional state, and anxiety.

🌀 Participants who microdosed the placebo (in the control arm) reported improvements from mood, energy, creativity, emotional state, and anxiety, at a slightly lower rate than those receiving an active microdose.

🌀 Expectation bias potentially increases the chances that people will have improved outcomes with medications, placebos, and microdosing psychedelic medicines.

CHAPTER 11

HOW DO I DISCUSS MICRODOSING WITH MY HEALTHCARE PROVIDER?

So, you think microdosing might be right for you. Like any major lifestyle change, it is recommended that you have a discussion with your medical professional (primary care provider [PCP] and/or psych provider) about this decision. In this chapter I discuss how to talk with your healthcare provider and address any concerns that they may have. Later, in Chapter 14, "Medications and Microdosing," I discuss how your healthcare provider can support those looking to microdose.

I encourage you to bring this guidebook with you to your appointment when you plan to discuss microdosing, so your provider can review Part 2 of this book and the source material. Don't become discouraged if your provider doesn't want to give you an answer the first time you bring up microdosing. Many do not know too much about microdosing, and it may seem "extreme" to them at first. Allow them to take time to learn more about it; you want them to be able to digest the information and make informed decisions about your healthcare.

Remember, one of the main reasons I took the time to write this guidebook was to help share information on microdosing in one handy package. To the best of my knowledge, there are no other books available for both individuals and healthcare professionals about microdosing. My goal is to bridge the gap between people who want to microdose and their healthcare providers. After exploring microdosing and one's individual needs more in depth, both parties can then make informed, collaborative healthcare decisions.

STARTING A CONVERSATION ABOUT MICRODOSING

First, I don't recommend you go into such a conversation automatically expecting your provider to be completely against the idea of microdosing. Also, you shouldn't avoid discussing microdosing because you think you know what they will say. Many healthcare providers are starting to learn about the benefits that psychedelics could provide, but they may not advertise it. Serendipitously, the first-ever patient I met as a psychiatric mental health provider asked me if I knew anything about microdosing for depression.

Due to licensure concerns, personal practice insurances, and the stigmas still associated with psychedelics, most medical professionals will not bring up these discussions themselves. Just like discussions about smoking, alcohol use, and drug use, psychedelics can be approached in a frank and open conversation. Don't worry, I will provide you with some basic information to reference that describes the substance's safety profiles and how you may be able to collaboratively mitigate risks.

You can also make your healthcare provider aware that Part 2 of this guidebook provides details about where they may access information themselves and discover professional organizations that provide accredited educational opportunities to learn more. Many of these accredited education programs were written by healthcare providers for providers. Psychedelic-aware providers are out there, and our numbers are increasing.

Like I said, bring this book with you to your appointment. Share your questions, concerns, and thoughts. Write some of the questions you have for your healthcare provider in the blank pages provided. Take notes. Go into your appointment prepared to ask questions.

WHAT SHOULD MY MEDICAL PROVIDER AND I DISCUSS?

One important piece of information to understand is that all medical professionals base their practice on up-to-date research, evidence-based practices, and personal/professional experiences. Unfortunately, research may come out quicker than your provider is aware of it. Therefore, healthcare providers must continue their educational growth and maintain continued education throughout their careers. Individual types of continuing education are based on their specialty and field of study; psychedelic medicines are still considered new and experimental since they are still classified as Schedule I substances.

A great place for providers to start is to review "Human Hallucinogen Research: Guidelines for Safety" located in Chapter 13 in Part 2 of this guidebook. Here, they may become familiar with the standard medical clearances necessary for participation in psychedelic research, which may help them feel more at ease.

Here is a list of conditions, disorders, plus medications you may currently be taking that you might want to discuss with your provider. Each is discussed at length in the relevant chapters cited.

- **Psychiatric Considerations**—Please refer to "Psychiatric Considerations and Microdosing" on "Psychiatric Considerations and Microdosing" on page 144.

- **Bipolar Disorders**—Please refer to "Bipolar Disorders and Microdosing" on page 146.

- **Psychosis and Thought Disorders**—Please refer to "Psychosis/History of Psychosis and Microdosing" on page 145.

- **Medical/Cardiac Conditions**—Please refer to "Physiological Considerations and Microdosing" on page 139. Here I will specifically discuss medical considerations including cardiac concerns, urinary

considerations, breastfeeding, cluster headaches/
migraines, and serotonin syndrome.

The following can all be found in Chapter 14, "Medications and
Microdosing."

🌀 **Antidepressant Medications–** Please refer to
"Antidepressants and Microdosing" on page 149. Here
I will specifically discuss SSRI/SNRI medications, MAOIs,
tricyclic medications, miscellaneous other antidepressant
medications, and serotonin syndrome.

🌀 **Antipsychotic Medications**—Please refer to
"Antipsychotic Medications and Microdosing" on
page 155. Here I discuss first-generation and second-
generation antipsychotic medications.

🌀 **Anxiolytic Medications**—Please refer to "Anxiolytics
and Microdosing" on page 158. Here I specifically
discuss various classes of anxiolytic medications including
benzodiazepines, sympatholytics, antihistamines,
gabapentinoid medications, and Silexan (lavender oil
supplements).

🌀 **Mood Stabilizers**—Please refer to "Medications for
Bipolar Disorder and Microdosing" on page 166. Here I
specifically discuss mood stabilizers including lamotrigine,
lithium, and valproic acid.

🌀 **Psychostimulant Medications**—Please refer to
"Psychostimulants and Microdosing" on page 155.

🌀 **Pain Medications**—Please refer to "Pain Medications
and Microdosing" on page 163. Here I discuss various
medications including analgesics, gabapentinoids, opiates,
and tramadol.

PART 2:
THE PROVIDER'S HANDBOOK

CHAPTER 12

AUTHOR'S NOTE TO CLINICIANS

Author's Note: By this point in the guidebook, you should have a solid grasp on what microdosing is, how it might help you, and how to go about doing it. These next chapters will cover some of the topics and information a little deeper than what is generally necessary for the average person looking to microdose. I'll share more in-depth information for healthcare providers who want to learn more and provide specific information on how to support individuals looking to microdose. As such, this information is more clinically based. I have cited the source material, and in the case the results are not conclusive, I have given a rationale for conclusions. This information should not dictate medical decisions; always use your own clinical judgment for your client's individual needs.

We need to remember that all individuals participate in treatments in hopes that they make some form of improvement. This active participation can lead to two unmeasurable factors. The first is an expectation bias. The second is an enhanced placebo effect. Both factors are important because they can lead to better outcomes. Your buy-in when patients seek your input into their decision to microdose is just as important as their buy-in when you prescribe medications or recommend treatment options. Neither the role of you or your patients is any more important in this situation. Optimal outcomes are achieved through active engagement in treatment. This therapeutic alliance and collaborative approach is crucial for care, and these points are almost more important than actual treatment for many conditions.

It is important to also consider the patient's individual journey of wellness and explore their motivations for seeking this as a treatment option. As clinicians, we should consider that if an individual is coming to us to discuss microdosing as a treatment option then they have probably started to explore what this means and what it entails. If they are having this dialogue, they are likely in the contemplative or early preparation stage of change.

If they are talking to you about such treatment, then they may be seeking your input and expertise on how to microdose safely and avoid potential drug interactions. Even if you are reading this because a patient handed you this guidebook and asked if microdosing is right for them, and you do not agree with this regimen due to political, sociological, or philosophical views, that is OK. But it's possible they may be looking for support and reassurance only—their decision may already be made.

Consider this and take an approach from the harm-reduction model. I know this may sound radical, but If you withhold information, even if that is simply reassurance, they may still follow through with microdosing, and an important moment of trust and rapport can be lost. If you feel uncomfortable answering their questions, you can refer them to someone else who is more knowledgeable about microdosing. Not giving information or shutting them down may cause more harm than necessary. *Remember: First, do no harm.*

How you approach the conversation and how open you are to the conversation is crucial. Any reaction that can come across as negative, condescending, or inaccurate could cause a significant barrier in your working relationship. I have heard many who have asked me for input because they do not want to talk to their provider about microdosing, are worried about their provider's reaction, are worried about the consequences of their working relationship moving forward, or do not want to have anything about microdosing in their medical record.

The last concern, not wanting it to be written in their record, may be motivated because of the stigma associated with psychedelics, long-term legal ramifications, and concerns of what may happen if others find out (e.g., their insurance company, other providers, family, etc.). Taking the initiative to have this discussion with a patient's provider is a huge step since it has been reported that less than 20 percent of the participants discussed microdosing with their provider before initiating a microdosing protocol (Lea et al. 2020b). Think of it this way: for every single patient who inquires about microdosing, there are four others who don't ask.

When patients do ask, here are some sample questions and concerns to help facilitate a dialogue. Mentally preparing for these questions may help you to gain an understanding into their motivations, treatment goals, and what you may want to say in response. As their clinician, you may already know some of their answers, but asking them would be great to not only build your clinical alliance but also help build rapport, trust, and understanding. This preparation may help to improve the patient's expectations and the enhanced placebo effects discussed earlier.

In the case of patients who are considering microdosing, exploring their individual motivations is key.

⚘ Why does the client feel microdosing may be beneficial?

- ○ Common answers may include numerous failed medication trials, poor response to antidepressants, intolerable side effects from conventional treatments/medications.

⚘ Does the client have a predominantly depressed presentation with a diagnosis of bipolar II?

- ○ Have you both been attempting to avoid serotonergic antidepressants in fear they contribute to an induction of manic symptoms?

⚘ Does the client have an aversion to pharmaceuticals and prefer to attempt holistic treatments or plant medicines?

⚘ We need to remember, if a patient is experiencing intolerable side effects, then often they may choose to stop their medications completely (even without telling you).

At this point, what are we really treating and why are they coming back to see you?

🌀 Clinicians who may not consider the patient's preferences may contribute to the patient experiencing a "nocebo" effect from any treatment modality. Buy-in is key!

Fundamentally, do clinicians need to be completely hung up on the fact that patient improvements may not be fully due to a pharmaceutical intervention, or should we take more of a Machiavellian approach? By that, I mean "the ends justify the means."

One topic of education to discuss should be related to the legality of these psychedelic substances. It may be important to explain that even if many of the psychedelic substances are decriminalized in your municipality, they are still illegal at the federal level. This topic is explored in Chapter 9, "The Legality of Microdosing."

CHAPTER 13

SPECIAL CONSIDERATIONS

Briefly discussed in Part 1 of this guidebook, classic psychedelic medicines are generally well tolerated and considered safe, but there are a couple of medical and psychiatric conditions that should be taken into consideration before an individual decides to begin a microdosing regimen. In this chapter I explain general safety protocols that researchers and those who use psychedelic medicines follow and how to best support our patients.

HUMAN HALLUCINOGEN RESEARCH: GUIDELINES FOR SAFETY

The Human Hallucinogen Research: Guidelines for Safety was written to describe some of the unique effects and potential adverse reactions participants may experience in clinical trials utilizing psychedelic substances (Johnson, Richards, and Griffiths 2008). The goal of this publication was to describe some of the challenges encountered in psychedelic research and help improve safety for those working with these substances. Classic hallucinogenic substances (including psilocybin and LSD) have been shown to have low physiological risks and be free from potential neurotoxic effects, while leaving most of the troublesome or noxious effects to be psychological in nature, not physical (Johnson et al. 2008).

These preliminary guidelines are currently accepted as gold-standard practices for high-dose psychedelic research and are still utilized in research conducted to this day, although some restrictions are less rigid as we have learned more. Currently there are no guidelines or significant research regarding safety concerns for microdose amounts of psychedelic substances. Many of the conclusions regarding safety come from either the early research conducted to understand the effects of low-dose psychedelics, data collected from low-dose administration of psychedelics (often used as a placebo in many larger dose research studies), or data extrapolated from results conducted in high-dose psychedelic research.

Since these safety guidelines are the basis for macrodoses of psychedelics, it would seem reasonable this may be a good place to start for individuals wanting to microdose.

PHYSICAL ASSESSMENT

According to the human hallucinogenic research guidelines, participants should be in good physical health and able to tolerate the physiological changes that psychedelics produce. The guidelines encourage that participants should be assessed and deemed in good physical health by obtaining a routine workup that includes:

- Medical history and physical exam (to assess current physical status and past medical history)
- Twelve-lead ECG (specifically for cardiac history or concerns)
- Standard labs (e.g., CBC, CMP, urinalysis)
- Negative pregnancy test (practicing safe/effective birth-control methods)

SPECIFIC EXCLUSIONS

The Human Hallucinogen Research: Guidelines for Safety describe some physical and psychological conditions that should be considered to possibly exclude one from being a good candidate for participation in research using psychedelic substances, or, in our case, *using* psychedelic substances. The most significant physical condition is hypertension.

Due to the moderate increases in the cardiovascular system that result from high-dose classic hallucinogens, those with systolic blood pressures >140 mmHg or diastolic >90 mmHg averaged over four assessments over two days are excluded from participation in drug trials.[5]

Psychiatric conditions such as psychosis, schizophrenia, and bipolar disorders may also exclude candidates from using psychedelic substances, per these guidelines for safety. We'll look at those in the "Psychiatric Considerations" section, following "Physiological Considerations."

PHYSIOLOGICAL CONSIDERATIONS AND MICRODOSING

Apart from the concerns discussed in *The Human Hallucinogen Research: Guidelines for Safety*, which focus more specifically on macrodoses of psychedelic medicines, there are some specific concerns for microdoses of psychedelics. These relate to the fact that unlike macrodoses, where dosing occurs infrequently and then it's over, microdosing causes chronic, intermittent stimulation of serotonin receptors and the cascade of effects that result from this stimulation. These are broken up into physical and psychological concerns later in this chapter.

CARDIAC CONCERNS IN MICRODOSING

Classic psychedelics have been long known to have stimulating effects on the cardiovascular system (Isbell 1959) and cardiac concerns such as hypertension have been exclusionary

---

5. Note: The authors asserted that these limits may be reconsidered in future studies. Since its original publication, several studies have changed their exclusion criteria. Regarding microdosing, there are some specific cardiac concerns that will be discussed in depth, just up ahead in the next section.

conditions for many psychedelic studies, as noted above. As of this book's release date, there isn't any published research showing safety considerations for microdose amounts of psychedelics that focus on cardiac conditions (e.g., hypertension or dysrhythmias).

Specific to microdosing, there some hypothetical cardiac concerns to note. The first is the general concern that all individuals with cardiac conditions should avoid stimulants. The second is a more specific concern that relates to the actions of a previously undescribed serotonin receptor, the 5-HT2B receptors.

STIMULATION OF THE 5-HT2B RECEPTORS

In the recently published *Handbook of Medical Hallucinogens* (2021), board-certified psychiatric pharmacists Kelan Thomas and Benjamin Malcolm briefly describe potential complications of microdosing psychedelic substances related to cardiac concerns. These hypothetical concerns are only related to microdosing and unresearched to this point. The question is based on what the long-term effects may be of stimulating the 5-HT2B receptors, which does not occur with the administration of high-dose psychedelics. Microdosing may stimulate these receptors with each administration, which may then cause physiological changes.

Chronic stimulation of the 5-HT2B receptors has been shown to result in cardiac concerns such as valvular heart disease (VHD), cardiac hypertrophy, and abnormal mitochondrial functioning. These effects have been found in other medications such as fenfluramine, one-half of the popular anti-obesity medication fen-phen in the early 1990s, antimigraine medications ergotamine and methysergide, and antiparkinson medications cabergoline and pergolide. Like these medications, both psilocybin and LSD have been found to have an affinity to the serotonin 5-HT2B receptors, but it is not known how much activation of the 5-HT2B receptors is necessary to develop side effects such as VHD, nor is it known if microdosing psychedelics activate these receptors enough to cause these effects. Despite the lack of published research affirming or discrediting microdosing's effect on 5-HT2B receptors and the potential to cause VHD, renowned neuropsychopharmacologist David Nutt did publicly announce on Twitter in 2020 that he has conducted unpublished research asserting "DAVE Nicholls (sic) and I modelled this a few years ago and found it unlikely that even repeated microdosing would influence the 2b receptor enough. @Drug_Science". Understandably, this is only one claim by one person, but it may help ease clinicians' worries.

Ultimately, if individuals decide to microdose, the safest approach is to consider Thomas's (2019) recommendation: "Based on this limited evidence, a shorter duration of microdosing (weeks to months) with longer breaks would likely be lower risk than a longer duration of dosing without any breaks for years."

It would be worth noting that the primary symptoms associated with VHD are chest pain, lightheadedness, and shortness of breath, but there are also some who report never having any recognizable physical symptoms. VHD can be easily ruled out by the absence of a heart murmur during a physical exam by a PCP, but the "gold standard" to detect valvular damages would be an echocardiogram ("echo").

URINARY CONSIDERATIONS IN MICRODOSING

One of the lesser-known effects of psychedelic use is the impact on the ureters, which connect the kidneys to the urinary bladder. Stimulation of the 5-HT2A receptors can cause tissues in the ureters to become more fibrous and constrict, which may include a complete closure. These effects are dose dependent, but the dose amount is also unknown, and once the stimulating agent is removed from the body, the effects should resolve themselves. Needing actual medical intervention is extremely rare. The chance of this happening can be further decreased by avoiding daily microdosing, which allows more time for substances to metabolize out of the body.

BREASTFEEDING AND MICRODOSING

Psilocin and psilocybin are eliminated through the kidneys, most of which occurs within the first three hours after oral ingestion and completely within twenty-four hours (Hasler et al. 2002). Unlike psilocybin, LSD is metabolized through the liver as the potentially inactive metabolite 2-oxo-3-hydroxy-LSD (Dolder et al. 2017) and is nearly completely excreted between four to six hours (Passie et al. 2008). Even in macrodoses, due to the potency of LSD, only very small amounts (micrograms) are ingested. Microdoses are even smaller. Due to the quick metabolism of classic psychedelics, microdosing can be done while breastfeeding. James Fadiman asserts that if individuals wait at least six hours between microdosing and breastfeeding, there shouldn't be any reason for concern (Morski 2020). In addition, there is no evidence that either substance is eliminated through breast milk.

Ideally, women would eliminate all substances that may raise concern while breastfeeding, but there is no research supporting or disproving these safety concerns.

CLUSTER HEADACHES/MIGRAINES AND MICRODOSING

Unlike the other symptoms mentioned, dosing recommendations and frequency may be specifically prescribed for cluster headaches. This is because individuals with cluster headaches (described as experiencing two or more periods of daily headaches for a month or more) have been found to have longer periods of remission as a result of microdosing tryptamines—classic psychedelic substances such as psilocybin and LSD are within this class of medications (Sicuteri 1963).

There are historical reports describing the use of LSD specifically as an effective treatment for cluster headaches and migraines. In one such study, the authors assert that "LSD is a good migraine prophylactic agent in non-hallucinogenic doses, such as 0.1–0.2 mg/kg [i.e., 7–15 mcg] (Sicuteri 1977, 57). In separate studies, researchers found that taking three microdoses of psychedelics, with a five-day interval between doses, had the best effect for headache prophylaxis (Karst et al. 2010; Sewell et al. 2006).

These effects are believed to be partly due to the action psychedelic substances have on the serotonin 5-HT1D receptors, not 5-HT2A receptors, which is a similar mechanism of action for other medications commonly prescribed for chronic headache and migraine relief (e.g., Imitrex/sumatriptan) (Fookes 2021). Unfortunately for those suffering these conditions, there are not many of these substances available on the market. But research has shown those who have not found adequate relief from conventional pharmaceuticals may find it from micro-dosing psychedelics, with minimal safety concerns (Andersson et al. 2017; Sewell et al. 2006).

Currently, there are Phase 2 clinical trials exploring LSD for the treatment of cluster headaches, but not at dosages that are classified as a microdose. Moving ahead, the potential implications of successful Phase 2 and Phase 3 clinical trials are huge. If researchers can prove statistically significant improvements from psychedelic medicines and gain FDA approval, this would open the floodgates for more changes, including proving that these substances should be removed from DEA Schedule I substances, a class which is reserved for drugs that are considered the most dangerous (defined as addictive and without medicinal qualities). Other implications of rescheduling are increased access and potentially allowing medical providers to prescribe these medications for off-label indications.

SEROTONIN SYNDROME

Serotonin Syndrome is discussed thoroughly in the next chapter, "Medications and Microdosing."

PSYCHIATRIC CONSIDERATIONS AND MICRODOSING

Contemporary psychedelic research has cautiously excluded individuals who have a current or past history of schizophrenia or a psychotic disorder, or those with a first-degree family member with those conditions. One thing to consider is that most psychedelic research is conducted using large or macrodoses, and only a small fraction comes from low or microdose amounts. Further, most of the low-dose research was completed in the past and was not in accordance with today's standards.

PSYCHOSIS/HISTORY OF PSYCHOSIS AND MICRODOSING

Classic psychedelics/hallucinogens have been found to potentially provoke onset of a prolonged psychosis (defined as lasting longer than intended after ingestion of a substance), which can persist for days or even months (Strassman 1984). The chance of this occurring is actually quite rare (0.8 out of 1,000) and, incidentally, less common than someone participating in outpatient psychotherapy, which was found to be 1.8 per 1,000 participants (Cohen 1960).

It is theorized those who have experienced prolonged psychotic reactions after taking psychedelic substances may have had a genetic predisposition to experiencing that reaction. Research reflects this correlation but cannot prove causation. It is not clearly understood if the psychotic reaction would have occurred as early as it was experienced, or if the psychotic break would have ever occurred whatsoever (Grinspoon and Bakalar 1979; Strassman 1984). As a result, *The Human Hallucinogen Research: Guidelines for Safety* proposed exclusion of participants who have personal and/or family histories of psychotic disorders. Like cardiac conditions, these restrictions have slowly eased back, allowing more research for individuals with these conditions.

BIPOLAR DISORDERS AND MICRODOSING

Due to exclusion of individuals with a history of bipolar disorder in psychedelic research, it is not entirely clear what the effects of microdosing may have on individuals. In time we should learn more about this relationship as exclusionary criteria becomes less restrictive. For now, it seems reasonable to approach microdosing and bipolar disorders similar to how one may approach standard antidepressant medications such as SSRIs or SNRIs and bipolar disorders, being mindful of potential side effects and the potential to induce mood instability. This is because psychedelics' mechanisms of action are through stimulation of the serotonin system, albeit through different pathways. It does seem reasonable that some unwanted complications could result, including the induction of manic symptoms or a full-blown manic episode, similar to the effect of SSRIs. Careful education should be provided, as well as a caution to observe changes in mood, especially during early phases of microdosing or when the individual may increase their dosages.

As of publication, there is a dearth of evidence showing a direct correlation between the use of serotonergic psychedelics, bipolar disorder, and the induction of manic episodes. In a case study published by Hendin and Penn (2021), they discuss these challenges and this lack of evidence. In that research, a twenty-one-year-old female, previously undiagnosed with bipolar disorder, appeared to have developed a manic episode (with psychotic features) that was seemingly induced by a macrodose of psilocybin. While the authors discuss macrodoses of psilocybin, there are some points to consider and then extrapolate as considerations for microdosing.

The patient had been previously treated with psychotherapy; fluoxetine, an SSRI medication; repetitive transcranial magnetic stimulation (rTMS); and adjunctive ketamine infusions, and she did not experience treatment-emergent mania secondary to either the SSRI medications nor the rTMS treatments, both of which have been shown to induce mania in some. But she did develop her first manic episode after ingesting a macrodose of psilocybin. Since SSRI medications and psychedelics have different mechanisms of action, this may be the reason the psilocybin induced mania and the SSRIs (and other medications) did not. Ideally, in time we will have a better understanding of these relationships.

Ultimately, knowing the risks of psychedelic medicine within those bipolar disorders would be immensely beneficial. I believe this is one segment of the population that may benefit the most from psychedelic medicines, in both macrodoses or microdoses, especially for those with a predominately depressed bipolar presentation, as the management of depression in individuals with bipolar disorder is notoriously difficult to manage by pharmacological methods.

Patients with a history of bipolar diagnoses who are interested in microdosing can mitigate risks and maximize results with safety planning, journaling, and having someone they know and trust help monitor their mood. Specific medication considerations for the management of bipolar disorder and microdosing are discussed more in-depth in the next chapter.

CHAPTER 14

MEDICATIONS AND MICRODOSING

This chapter is for the healthcare provider looking to support patients who want to learn more about microdosing and may have specific questions about potential medication interactions.

Regarding medications, there are numerous resources out there (many are anecdotal) but one reputable site (www .microdosingpsychedelics.com) is run by James Fadiman and Sophia Korb. This website is an updated list of medications and supplements from which users have reported experiencing no negative or adverse effects when taken while microdosing psychedelics. I want to share this because your patients may cite information that they have found on the web for themselves. I would caution this information may be from anecdotal observations only.

ANTIDEPRESSANTS AND MICRODOSING

Antidepressant medications, and how they differ from microdosing, were discussed briefly in Chapter 10, "Mental Health and Microdosing." Now I will explore more deeply the different types of antidepressant medications and some specific concerns regarding microdosing.

SSRIs/SNRIs AND MICRODOSING

SSRIs are the most common antidepressant medication, accounting for 80 percent of all such prescriptions. The primary mechanism of action for SSRI medications is achieved through blocking the reuptake of serotonin by the serotonin transporters (SERT). In the brain, this results in an increased amount of free serotonin within the synapses, which ideally results in an uplifting of mood, decreased anxiety, and improvements in distress tolerance. One of the effects that results from increasing serotonin in the brain is that the body will adjust. One such process is "down regulation," in which the number of serotonin receptors in the brain may decrease. Normally, this would not be a big deal, but when we consider taking serotonergic psychedelic substances, there may be fewer serotonin receptors for these substances to attach to.

Unfortunately, it's not completely clear how this affects microdosing. Based on one particular study (Bonson, Buckholtz, & Murphy 1996), many believe that psychedelic effects will be blocked. In that study, the reported effects from LSD macrodoses were significantly decreased in those who reported chronic SSRI administration prior to use. To date, there have not been any specific studies examining if this affects psilocybin. Many report no noticeable difference in effects from macrodoses of psilocybin with concurrent, chronic SSRI administration (Malcolm 2020). And, on the other hand, some have reported finding benefit from concurrent use, but that may be attributed to the placebo effect or something else. I wish I could give a better, more conclusive answer.

SEROTONIN SYNDROME

The second most popular question that many will ask regarding microdosing is "Will taking antidepressant medications with psychedelics cause serotonin syndrome?" To be clear, when I am referring to psychedelics in this sense, I am describing the classic (tryptamine) psychedelics (e.g., psilocybin and LSD), and not MAOI-containing psychedelics (e.g. ayahuasca) or ibogaine.

Serotonin syndrome, also known as serotonin toxicity, is a potentially life-threatening condition that is a diagnosis of exclusion, meaning in order for a diagnosis to be made, clinicians need to rule out other causes for the presentation as there isn't any single diagnostic test that can confirm the diagnosis. Serotonin syndrome is caused by the use of serotonergic medications and an overactivation of serotonin receptors, often as a result of taking numerous drugs (polypharmacy) that raise serotonin levels, such as a combination of serotonergic medications; for instance, antidepressant medications; complex drug interactions (often working on different mechanisms); or as a result from overdosing on these medications.

It's not entirely known how frequently serotonin syndrome occurs, because mild cases are often not reported or the presentations are attributed to other causes. The presentation of serotonin syndrome can range from mild symptoms to serious and life-threatening conditions and include symptoms of mild hypertension, tachycardia, increased sweating, dilation of the pupils, shivering, tremor, twitching, hyperreflexia, and hyperthermia. In severe cases individuals may present with severe hyperthermia, dramatic swings in pulse and blood pressure, delirium, and muscle rigidity. These severe cases can result in complications such as seizures, rhabdomyolysis (muscle breakdown and a release of proteins into the blood), renal failure, respiratory distress, coma, and death.

The good news is there have not been any documented cases of serotonin syndrome associated with classic psychedelics, singularly or with concurrent serotonin agonist medications (Koslow 2020; Malcolm 2019).

If you dig deep enough into the research, you may find a single case study alleging a correlation between psilocybin use and serotonin syndrome in three individuals (Suzuki 2016). Many have voiced criticisms of this publication and its lack of academic rigor as it is only published in Japanese (lacking official reprints in other languages), its references include hyperlinks to websites that are broken, the websites that worked did not describe anything about psilocybin and serotonin syndrome, and the other references gave only superficial information about psilocybin. Overall, this publication may best be discredited completely, but I mention it for full disclosure's sake. I have made attempts to contact the author of this paper to discuss the topic more thoroughly and have not received any correspondence in return.

Ben Malcolm (2021), "the Spirit Pharmacist," asserts that "The mechanism of psilocybin helps inform the safety profile: due to an inability to increase intrasynaptic serotonin as well as an inability to fully stimulate serotonin receptors the same way that serotonin itself would, there is little risk of overwhelming serotonin neurotransmission or for a truly life-threatening serotonin syndrome to occur—even when combined with other substances that can increase 5HT (e.g. SSRIs, MAOIs, MDMA)."

So, it appears that overall, the combination of SSRI/SNRI and classic psychedelics is probably safe, especially since the doses we are discussing are microdoses. At larger doses (full psychedelic trip), the combination is probably safe as well, but the psychedelic effects may be blunted (Koslow 2020; Malcolm 2021).

TRICYCLIC ANTIDEPRESSANTS (TCAs) AND MICRODOSING

Tricyclic antidepressants (e.g., Elavil/amitriptyline, Pamelor/nortriptyline, Anafranil/clomipramine) are less common now than other antidepressant medications, and their mechanisms of action are different from other antidepressant medications. TCAs work by blocking the reuptake of serotonin and norepinephrine at the receptor sites. TCAs are sometimes also prescribed for sleep or prophylactically to treat migraines and cluster headaches, which is why psychedelics may be effective as a treatment option for these conditions.

Chronic use of TCAs has been shown to potentiate the subjective effects of LSD (e.g., physiological, psychological, and hallucinatory reactions) in participants taking macrodoses (Bonson & Murphy 1996; Passie et al. 2008). Due to the similar reactions of psilocybin and LSD, this effect may be extrapolated to be similar from concurrent psilocybin use. But, there isn't any current literature confirming or discrediting this hypothesis if the psychedelic dosage is a microdose instead of a macrodose.

While I am not specifically recommending concurrent use of TCAs and microdosing, you may want to educate your patient to consider starting at the lower end of psychedelic dosing.

MAOIs AND MICRODOSING

Monoamine oxidase inhibitor (MAOI) antidepressant medications have a unique mechanism of action compared to SSRIs and TCAs, because they block the breakdown of neurotransmitters in the brain (serotonin, norepinephrine, and dopamine).

There are two types of MAOIs—MAOI-As and MAOI-Bs—and either type may block the effects of microdosing:

MAOI-As (e.g. Nardil, Parnate) have been found to potentially inhibit psychedelic effects of LSD in some, but it is not clear for psilocybin (Bonson & Murphy 1996).

MAOI-Bs (i.e., Emsam/selegiline) are thought to have a low risk for physical toxicity when used with LSD and psilocybin (Malcolm 2020).

OTHER ANTIDEPRESSANT MEDICATIONS

The following two drugs may interfere with psychedelics.

REMERON (MIRTAZAPINE) AND MICRODOSING

Remeron's mechanism of action is different from other antidepressants in that it blocks the 5-HT2A receptors, which means it is very likely to blunt psychedelic effects of both LSD and psilocybin (Gilman 2017). It is unclear how this would be affected by microdose amounts, but it's highly likely that it would negate the effects.

TRAZODONE AND MICRODOSING

The antidepressant medication Trazodone is commonly prescribed off-label for insomnia. Trazodone blocks the 5-HT2A receptors, which may disrupt effects for macrodoses of psychedelics (Gilman 2017). It is unclear how concurrent microdoses (psilocybin or LSD) and trazodone administration will result, but it may be advantageous to find alternatives if taking trazodone as needed (PRN) to facilitate sleep. Or just don't use it the night prior to microdose administration.

ANTIPSYCHOTIC MEDICATIONS FOR DEPRESSION

Sometimes people will take low-dose antipsychotic medications as augmenting agents for depression. For more information, please refer to the section "Antipsychotic Medications and Microdosing" just up ahead.

PSYCHOSTIMULANTS AND MICRODOSING

"Psychostimulants" are used generically in this guidebook to include medications such as Ritalin (methylphenidate), Adderall (amphetamine salts), and any of their various formulations. Concurrent microdosing and psychostimulant use causes increased activity in the cardiovascular system. There aren't any specific issues that occur from concurrent use, but I would caution patients that overuse or overstimulation from these medications may lead to sleep disturbances, increased anxiety, and the potential for increased chances of developing acute or prolonged psychotic reactions.

If patients decide to concurrently microdose while using psychostimulant medications, they should use caution, start slowly, and approach this similarly to microdosing while using other stimulating substances such as caffeine or energy drinks. You may want to explain that they may not need to use the psychostimulants while microdosing, or they may prefer to take some time between their microdose and psychostimulant medication.

ANTIPSYCHOTIC MEDICATIONS AND MICRODOSING

Antipsychotic medications can be summed up into two separate subcategories: first-generation antipsychotics (FGAs) and second-generation antipsychotics (SGAs). Each has different mechanisms of action. Antipsychotic medications may block microdosing effects completely, which will be further delineated in the following subsections.

I am not endorsing concurrent antipsychotic medications and microdosing, nor am I condoning anyone with a history of psychosis to microdose, but these questions may come up, and some may be taking antipsychotic medications for other reasons such as an adjunct for depression, nausea, or to promote sleep. One educational point to address with patients who may want to stop antipsychotic medications and begin a microdosing regimen is that sudden discontinuation and subsequent psychedelic medications may result in a "supersensitivity psychosis" due to the prolonged deactivation of the neuroreceptors, specifically 5-HT2A (Charron et al. 2015) and dopamine (D2) (Chouinard, et al. 2017). It may be reasonable to encourage the patient to take a break between stopping antipsychotics and beginning microdosing.

FIRST-GENERATION ANTIPSYCHOTICS (FGAs)

First-generation antipsychotics are the classic antipsychotic medications, which act by blocking the dopamine (D2) receptors. Some of these medications include Thorazine (chlorpromazine), Haldol (haloperidol), and Prolixin (fluphenazine). These medications may not actually fully block the effects of microdosing, depending on their mechanism of action on other receptors.

In one study, one participant reported he was still able to have the intended psychedelic effects after receiving Haldol (Vollenwider, et al. 1998). Due to this, individuals may be able to theoretically microdose while concurrently taking haloperidol.[6]

Unlike other FGAs, Thorazine (chlorpromazine) has been shown to have an effect on 5-HT2A receptors and to block psychedelic effects as a result (Keeler 1967). Theoretically, chlorpromazine would completely block the effects of microdosing.

SECOND-GENERATION ANTIPSYCHOTICS (SGAs)

Second-generation antipsychotics, also known as atypical antipsychotics, work by blocking the serotonin 5-HT2A receptor along with dopamine (D2) receptors (Sullivan et al. 2015). The blocking of these receptors should theoretically mitigate some, if not all of the psychedelic effects of high-dose psilocybin administration. It would then seem reasonable to conclude that the blocking of the 5-HT2A receptors may render concurrent use while microdosing completely ineffective, like FGA chlorpromazine.

Some of these medications include Zyprexa (olanzapine), Risperdal (risperidone), Geodon (ziprasidone), Seroquel (quetiapine), and Abilify (aripiprazole).

CONCLUSION OF ANTIPSYCHOTIC MEDICATIONS AND MICRODOSING

While taking antipsychotic medications and microdosing may not seem like an ideal choice for patients, it might be advantageous to gain a better understanding of why they are

---

6. This is also why haloperidol is not an ideal choice to give to someone who is acutely psychotic, secondary to psychedelic ingestion in an emergency situation.

taking these medications and together explore alternative treatment options.

Individuals taking antipsychotic medications who may still be good candidates for microdosing are those with unipolar depression, anxiety, insomnia, or PTSD, who are being prescribed antipsychotics off-label for these indications. For those taking antipsychotic medications for bipolar disorder, please refer to the information that was discussed more thoroughly in the previous chapter. Taking the time to discuss a taper, discontinuation, and reassuring that you are open to such discussions may lead to better patient outcomes and better rapport between you and your patient.

ANXIOLYTICS AND MICRODOSING

At first glance, it may seem counterintuitive to microdose while concurrently using anxiolytics, but there may be reasons to do so. Remember, one motivation to microdose is to decrease medication or drug use, and microdosing may be part of this plan (if previously prescribed). In addition, anxiolytic medications may help for exacerbation of acute or breakthrough anxiety, similar to using these medications as adjunct medications for a newly established medication regimen. If microdosing does cause increased incidence of anxiety, encouraging a decreased microdosed amount may be warranted. Ideally, once an optimum dose is established, individuals may not need to use anxiolytic medications as often, but until then, there are options.

BENZODIAZEPINES AND MICRODOSING

While benzodiazepines' (e.g., Ativan/lorazepam, Klonopin/clonazepam, Xanax/alprazolam) mechanisms of action are not on the serotonin 5-HT2A receptors, in high-dose psychedelic use, benzodiazepines are known to blunt or block the psychedelic effects. Yet there is no clear or conclusive evidence of these effects at this time.

Per the human hallucination guidelines, benzodiazepines are recommended to be available for acute and dangerous reactions due to high-dose psychedelic administration since they can be used as an emergency medication to calm an individual (Griffiths et al. 2016). Benzodiazepines can be enacted as an "ejector seat and parachute" to remove the individual from a dangerous situation and slowly bring them back to a grounded state if an emergency arises.

While concurrent microdosing and the use of benzodiazepines is not dangerous, it may be advantageous to include discontinuing, or recommending benzodiazepine use only as needed (PRN), before starting a microdosing protocol. If that is not an ideal situation, collaboratively have a taper in mind; then once establishing the microdosing medicine's effects, you may consider discussing that microdosing may be used as part of a benzodiazepine taper plan, especially if the microdose regimen is helping to alleviate symptoms of chronic anxiety.

Due to microdosing's stimulant-like effects, microdosing may induce or exacerbate anxiety symptoms. Encouraging a lower microdose amount may help to diminish these effects. Other points to consider include letting the patient know that long-term benzodiazepine use can possibly contribute to physical dependency. Clinicians need to be mindful that sudden and rapid discontinuation of benzodiazepines could result in experiencing serious side effects, up to and including inducing seizure activity. Another discussion point to have with patients is to remind them that depending on your individual or institution's "controlled substance agreement," it is likely that microdosing will be a direct violation of this agreement. The biggest takeaway regarding concurrent microdosing and benzodiazepine use is that the safety profile looks to be good, but benzodiazepines may diminish intended effects for microdosing.

BUSPIRONE AND MICRODOSING

Buspar (buspirone) is an anxiolytic medication that is classified as a nonbenzodiazepine anxiolytic. Its mechanism of action is not completely known, but it is known to be a partial agonist of serotonin receptors (including 5-HT2A) and dopamine (D2) receptors. Since it does act on the 5-HT2A receptors, its concurrent use may block the effects of microdosing psychedelics (Pokorny et al. 2016). You may need to consider this and find alternative medications for your patient that do not block 5-HT2A receptors.

SYMPATHOLYTICS (ALPHA 2 AGONISTS AND BETA BLOCKERS) AND MICRODOSING

Another option for anti-anxiety medications that can be taken while microdosing are noncontrolled substances of the alpha 2 agonists or beta blocker families. Both clonidine (Hysek et al. 2012) and carvedilol (Hysek, Schmid, Rickli 2012)—each used to treat hypertension—were utilized as pre-treatment options for MDMA ("ecstasy") research and were found to be effective in decreasing physical symptoms of anxiety, through reducing hemodynamic effects and without altering subjective effects of MDMA. This is important because it shows even though the anxiolytic effects were felt, neither medication will block serotonin receptors, allowing for microdoses of psychedelics medications to still have their effects.

ANTIHISTAMINES AND MICRODOSING

Other options to consider for acute anxiety and microdosing are antihistamine medications such as hydroxyzine. Hydroxyzine does have a weak binding to 5-HT2A receptors, but it may not be strong enough to completely block its effect. There are numerous anecdotal reports that concurrent use of antihistamines with macrodoses of psychedelics does not negatively affect the psychedelic journey. In fact, some will prophylactically take diphenhydramine (Benadryl) with specific psilocybin-containing mushrooms (e.g., *Psilocybe azurescens*, *Psilocybe cyanescens*, and *Psilocybe subaeruginosa*) in an attempt to prevent symptoms of wood lover's paralysis (WLP). Reported symptoms of WLP include experiencing short-term muscle weakness, stiffness, or impaired motor functions, lasting for several hours after ingestion of these specific mushrooms. WLP is an underresearched phenomenon, and its exact cause is not known, but a common theme is all these mushrooms grow on wood, and not all individuals consistently experience WLP.

GABAPENTIN AND PREGABALIN AND MICRODOSING

Clinicians may also consider the off-label use of gabapentin or pregabalin for acute anxiety when patients are concurrently microdosing. Discussed in "Pain Medications and Microdosing," these options have anxiolytic properties and will not interfere with psychedelic medicine's mechanism of action. To note, pregabalin does have slightly better evidence for its anxiolytic effects compared to gabapentin, and pregabalin is approved for the treatment of generalized anxiety disorder (GAD) by the European Medicines Agency.

SILEXAN (LAVENDER OIL SUPPLEMENT) AND MICRODOSING

The last option to consider for the management of acute anxiety is actually a non-pharmacological agent: lavender oil supplements. Two of the main terpenoid constituents, linalool and linalyl acetate, are thought to produce their anxiolytic effects through inhibition of calcium channels, reduction of activity at the 5-HT1A receptors, and increased parasympathetic tone (Malcolm and Tallian 2017). The advantages of lavender oil are its lack of tolerance and abuse potential, it does not cause sedation, and it does not have any potential for producing withdrawal syndromes. These benefits are unlike conventional anxiolytic pharmaceuticals such as benzodiazepines, chronic SSRI/SNRI administration, and hydroxyzine.

Sold in Germany under the brand name Silexan, lavender oil supplements are available in the US as the over-the-counter dietary supplement CalmAid. Lavender oil supplements are available in 80 mg gel capsules and are recommended for either daily or twice-a-day dosing. Lavender oil supplements have been found to be more effective for anxiety compared to placebo, not inferior to daily dosing of lorazepam 0.5 mg daily for anxiety, and better at managing anxiety compared to placebo or paroxetine (an SSRI).

Lastly, the biggest side effect reported by lavender oil users has been described as the "not so unpleasant" lavender burps after oral ingestion. This may be an inexpensive, low-risk, high-reward option to consider recommending to patients, especially without adding another pharmacological agent, helping individuals to maintain natural treatment alternatives.

PAIN MEDICATIONS AND MICRODOSING

Briefly discussed in Chapter 6, "Microdosing Physical and Mental Health," serotonergic agonists have been shown to have anti-inflammatory properties. Early research has shown psychedelics, specifically microdosing psychedelics, are effective in reducing pain sensations in individuals and will be explored more thoroughly in the future. There is of course the added benefit psychedelics have over many conventional methods of pain management—serotonergic psychedelics are not addictive and there may not be any long-term complications resulting from their use.

"Pain medication" is the blanket term for any medication used to decrease perceived pain or pain sensations, and these range from analgesics to opiates to antidepressants to certain anticonvulsants such as gabapentin. Each type of "pain medication" needs to be addressed separately.

ANALGESICS AND MICRODOSING

For the purpose of this guidebook I will lump together generically various analgesics such as over-the-counter (OTC) aspirin, acetaminophen, and NSAIDs (e.g., ibuprofen).

There have not been any documented contraindications for concurrent use with microdosing, and they have been allowed for use in numerous psychedelic protocols.

GABAPENTINOIDS AND MICRODOSING

Gamma-aminobutyric acid, or GABA, is another neurotransmitter that has the role of sending chemical messages throughout the nervous system, including the brain. GABA is also involved in regulating communication between brain cells. GABA's role is to inhibit or reduce neural activity. Increasing GABA results in decreased pain, anxiety, and stress responses.

Gabapentinoids are a group of chemically similar medications that are often used off-label for numerous indications (such as neuropathic pain, anxiety, or sleep). Neurontin (gabapentin) and closely related Lyrica (pregabalin) both work in the GABA system, similar to anxiolytics such as benzodiazepines described earlier. As such, they may blunt psychedelic effects. These medications, like benzodiazepines, may cause dependence, and chronic administration of higher doses could lead to withdrawal if stopped suddenly (or seizures if being taken for a seizure disorder). There are no published studies exploring concurrent gabapentinoid medications and psychedelics. Extrapolated from the information mentioned in the benzodiazepine section, concurrent use may be theoretically safe, but you may want to address long-term plans with your patients.

OPIATES AND MICRODOSING

Opiates are any medications that bind with the μ (mu) opiate receptors. Since activation occurs at the opiate receptors, they do not act on the serotonin receptors (specifically 5-HT2A).

Theoretically, concurrent use should not pose a significant issue, but opiate medications (like all CNS depressants) have been shown to potentially blunt psychedelic effects in macrodose amounts. It is not understood if this also occurs at microdosing amounts. Patient education regarding chronic administration of opioids and rapid discontinuation leading to withdrawal symptoms should always be discussed.

TRAMADOL AND MICRODOSING

Tramadol is an opioid pain medication that also affects the serotonergic and noradrenergic systems. Tramadol specifically targets the serotonin 5-HT2C receptors (not 5-HT2A like classic psychedelics), which means it will not block the effects of microdosing. In addition, tramadol also increases serotonin levels through blocking postsynaptic reuptake of serotonin (and norepinephrine), similar to how SSRI/SNRI medications work. Concurrent use of tramadol and other serotonergic SSRI/SNRI medications has been associated with inducing serotonin syndrome (Beakley et al. 2015), but as discussed in "Antidepressants and Microdosing" on page 149, there are no known incidences of concurrent use of tramadol and microdosing leading to serotonin syndrome. In addition to the previously mentioned effects, tramadol has been shown to reduce the seizure threshold and induce seizures in some individuals—these seizures seem not to be related to inhibition of serotonin reuptake, distinctly different than seizures resulting from serotonin syndrome.

MEDICATIONS FOR BIPOLAR DISORDER AND MICRODOSING

Described in the previous chapter, the use of psychedelic substances is notoriously under-researched for individuals with bipolar disorder. The standard course of treatment for the different types of bipolar disorder is monotherapy or concurrent use of mood stabilizers, including the off-label use of antiepileptic medications and/or antipsychotic therapies.

MOOD STABILIZERS AND MICRODOSING

A recent publication entitled "Classic Psychedelic Coadministration with Lithium, but not Lamotrigine..." (Nayak et al. 2021) discussed various medications commonly used to treat bipolar disorders taken concurrently with macrodoses of classic psychedelics. The authors analyzed reports from three of the most common websites that collect and discuss psychedelic use (Erowid.org, Shroomery.org, and Reddit.com). Admittedly, these online reports are considered a low quality of evidence by scientific standards, but, unfortunately, it's all that's available at this time. Most of the information gained for their analysis was centered around lithium and lamotrigine. Other medications were mentioned (valproic acid sixteen times, carbamazepine eight times, and oxcarbazepine nine times), but the researchers felt this was not enough information to fully analyze the results. Each medication modality is discussed separately below.

LITHIUM AND MICRODOSING

Lithium, a mood stabilizer, is considered the "gold standard" treatment for bipolar disorder, for both its treatment of acute mania and prevention of relapse, and as an adjunct treatment to antidepressant therapy. The mechanisms of action for lithium are not entirely understood, and there is limited research showing how lithium interacts with psychedelic medicines. When lithium is taken in conjunction with macrodoses of LSD, some have reported experiencing increased psychedelic effects as a result (Bonson & Murphy 1996). These results may be extrapolated to include psilocybin, but there is no published data to support nor discredit the hypothesis.

In the article mentioned on page 166, "Classic Psychedelic Coadministration ..." (2021), Nayak et al. describe that individuals reporting concurrent classic psychedelic use with lithium therapy also describe having experienced intensified psychedelic effects, experiencing a "bad trip," and other more significant effects such as experiencing a seizure (47 percent) or needing to seek medical attention (39 percent). Only 8 percent of lithium users reported having a neutral experience.

The effect of concurrent lithium use and microdosing psychedelics is unknown. Some have reported microdosing while taking lithium without any untoward effects, and some have reported increased dizziness. Overall, concurrent use of lithium and microdosing is not recommended, but if your patients are determined to attempt this, it may be advantageous to encourage them to start microdosing at the lower end of the spectrum in an attempt to mitigate risks or minimize unwanted side effects (including seizures).

DEPAKOTE (VALPROIC ACID) AND MICRODOSING
Valproic acid, an antiepileptic medication, is often used for mood stabilization. Depakote is believed to work by affecting GABA levels. There are no known studies showing what may

occur with concurrent use with psychedelics in macrodose or microdose amounts. As such, it may be advantageous to start dosing low and slow when adding a microdosing regimen. In the future, it may be beneficial to explore these medications' concurrent use due to valproic acid's application for those with head injuries or poor impulse control.

LAMICTAL/LAMOTRIGINE AND MICRODOSING

Lamotrigine, also an antiepileptic medication, is often used as a mood stabilizer in psychiatry. Unlike other medications of the same category, lamotrigine is thought to work on the glutamate system. Unlike adverse events reported by lithium users when taken concurrently with classic psychedelics, described above, lamotrigine has been shown to be well tolerated when used in conjunction with classic psychedelics, and no one reported having experienced seizures or other adverse medical events resulting from concurrent use (Nayak et al. 2021). In addition, due to the length of time it takes to start or restart lamotrigine, it may be best to encourage individuals to continue lamotrigine during their microdosing regimen.

CHAPTER 15

EDUCATIONAL INFORMATION AND PROFESSIONAL ORGANIZATIONS

Here is a list of professional organizations and educational opportunities for healthcare professionals.

PROFESSIONAL ORGANIZATIONS

MULTIDISCIPLINARY ASSOCIATION OF PSYCHEDELIC STUDIES (MAPS): Founded in 1986, MAPS is the first organization founded with the goal to further education and understanding of psychedelic substances. MAPS has been an active proponent and participant in psychedelic research.

From their website: We are a 501(c)(3) nonprofit research and educational organization developing medical, legal, and cultural contexts for people to benefit from the careful uses of psychedelics and marijuana.

Website: https://maps.org

PSYCHEDELIC MEDICINE ASSOCIATION (PMA): Launched 2020, it is the first association for psychedelic practitioners. It has lots of information on psychedelics and health concerns.

It also has a podcast to stay up to date on information, a database for providers, and links to educational opportunities.

From their website: The Psychedelic Medicine Association is a society of physicians, therapists, and healthcare professionals looking to advance their education on the therapeutic uses of psychedelic medicines. We provide you with education and informational tools to help you feel confident to discuss psychedelic medicines with your patients. Create your professional profile and connect with like-minded health professionals as well as the organizations shaping the psychedelic industry.

Website: https://psychedelicmedicineassociation.org

OPENURSES: A not-yet-fully recognized (as of publication) professional organization.

From their website: The Organization of Psychedelic and Entheogenic Nurses (OPENurses) represents nurses, at all levels of training, who work with patients utilizing therapeutic psychedelic medicines. We exist to establish best practices; clearly define appropriate care in psychedelic sessions; elucidate a code of ethics and conduct; advocate for the full inclusion of nurses in psychedelic therapy; provide continuing education related to psychedelic therapy; and provide a place for professional networking.

Website: https://www.openurses.org

INTERNATIONAL ASSOCIATION OF PSYCHEDELIC NURSES (IAPN): A not-yet-fully recognized (as of publication) professional organization for nurses who also are interested in psychedelic medicines. The website has links for education and a database of nurses who are interested in psychedelics and can be contacted for more information.

From their website: Our mission is to promote increased global awareness and education on the topic of psychedelic medicines and to utilize the latest research in developing safe standards of nursing practice within an emerging field of study. Our mission is to aid every person in achieving safe, desirable outcomes when recovering from illness.

Website: https://www.psychedelicnursing.org

EDUCATIONAL PROGRAMS

PSYCHEDELICS TODAY: There are various courses for free and at a cost. The hallmark course "Navigating Psychedelics: For Clinicians and Therapists" is available on the website in either a self-guided format or as an interactive classroom. Offered at various times throughout the year, it's available for contact hours for professionals.

This course is a great resource for any medical or professional, especially, doctors, nurses, social workers, therapists, and other clinicians. I believe in this course. Not only have I taken it, but I have also contributed to the course. I also offer a course specifically for nurses on their website.

Psychedelics Today also has a great podcast published weekly to help you stay up-to-date on information regarding psychedelics.

Website: https://psychedelicstoday.com

PSYCHEDELIC.SUPPORT: This educational program launched in early 2020 and provides in-depth educational opportunities on various psychedelic substances (for contact hours). I believe in this course as well, and I contributed to the course on psilocybin.

Psychedelic.Support's website contains a database to find psychedelic practitioners in your area.

Website: http://psychedelic.support

PSYCHEDELIC SCHOOL: Psychedelic School is a great resource for providers and people wanting to learn more about psychedelics in general. Psychedelic School is owned and operated by Dr. Ben Malcolm, PharmD (aka Spirit Pharmacist), and his wife, Shiri Malcolm Godasi, MA, who is an integration educator and consultant. Both are very influential in psychedelic circles and innovative in the knowledge they bring to this space.

Website: https://www.psychedelicschool.com

CALIFORNIA INSTITUTE OF INTEGRAL STUDIES (CIIS): This offers the first accredited course for medical professionals to become approved to work with psychedelics once they are legal.

Website: https://www.ciis.edu

USONA: Usona Institute conducts clinical and preclinical psilocybin research. They conduct training for facilitators for psilocybin research.

Website: https://www.usonainstitute.org

FURTHER READING

If you want to learn more, I encourage you to do some reading of your own. Besides the research listed in the references section, other great resources to start with include:

🌀 *Your Psilocybin Mushroom Companion: An Informative, Easy-to-Use Guide to Understanding Magic Mushrooms— From Tips and Trips to Microdosing and Psychedelic Therapy* by Michelle Janikian (Ulysses Press, 2019)

🌀 *How to Change Your Mind: What the New Science of Psychedelics Teaches Us About Consciousness, Dying, Addiction, Depression, and Transcendence* by Michael Pollan (Penguin Books, 2018)

🌀 *The Psychedelic Explorer's Guide: Safe, Therapeutic, and Sacred Journeys* by James Fadiman (Park Street Press, 2011)

🌀 *Chanterelle Dreams, Amanita Nightmares: The Love, Lore, and Mystique of Mushrooms* by Greg Marley (Chelsea Green Publishing, 2010)

🌀 *Psilocybin: Magic Mushroom Grower's Guide—A Handbook for Psilocybin Enthusiasts* by O. T. Oss and O. N. Oeric (Quick American Archives, 2E, 1993). This handbook is admittedly outdated but was written by the McKenna brothers, Terrence and Dennis under pseudonyms in 1976.

🌀 *Cannabis: A Handbook for Nurses* by Carey S. Clark (LWW; First North American edition, 2021; other editions available). A former professor and mentor of mine, who through her own unconventional path in nursing inspired me to follow my own holistic nursing journey and write this guidebook.

🌀 *American Trip: Set, Setting, and the Psychedelic Experience in the Twentieth Century* by Ido Hartogsohn (MIT Press, 2020). This book along with his other published work made me think outside the box and question approaches in conventional medicines (specifically antidepressants) and the power of the placebo effect.

🌀 *Feeling Good: The New Mood Therapy* by David Burns (William Morrow and Company, 1980). This publication has been reprinted numerous times and now there are over four million copies in print. This book has been clinically shown to help around 60 percent of those who read it to have reduction in their depressive symptoms, higher than those who received the usual care for depression (Naylor et al. 2010).

Dr. Burn's website has lots of great information for people to learn more.

Website: http://feelinggood.com

Link to Bipolar and Magic Mushrooms Study:

https://www.crestbd.ca/2020/10/10/mushrooms-bipolar-disorder

In a strict sense, only those vision-producing drugs that can be shown to have figured in shamanic or religious rites would be designated entheogens, but in a looser sense, the term could also be applied to other drugs, both natural and artificial, that induce alterations of consciousness similar to those documented for ritual ingestion of traditional entheogens (Ruck et al. 1979).

From that day forward, I have been mindful of having faith in psychedelic medicine, allowing it to help guide my professional practice and jumping on board with projects that involve it. I am glad I have. Having faith in the process has allowed me to work on some amazing projects and learn so much more about these sacred substances. If you would have told me just three years ago when I treated the gentleman who presented psychotic from the Penis Envy mushrooms that I would be not only advocating, but also educating on their many benefits, I wouldn't have believed you. Nor could I ever in my wildest imagination think that we would be at the point that many cities and municipalities around the United States would be, decriminalizing these substances or moving toward the use as legitimate medicines. The movement is charging forward, like the mycological network below the soil. I guess maybe we all need to have a little faith in the way the mushroom is guiding us.

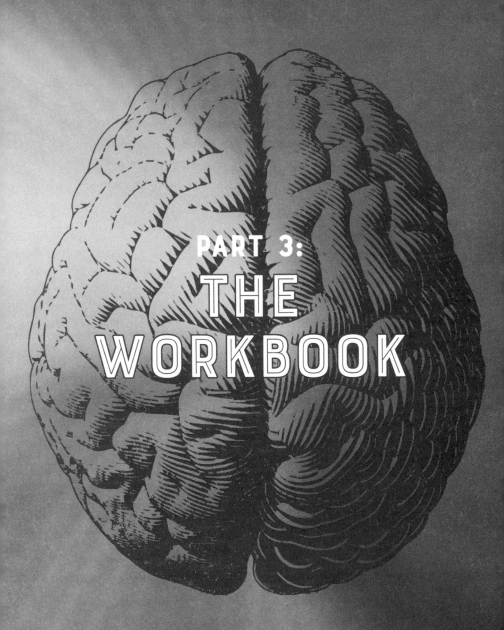

PART 3:
THE WORKBOOK

HANDS-ON TOOLS AND ACTIVITIES

Welcome to Part 3 of *The Microdosing Guidebook*—the workbook portion of the book. In this section, you will discover more tools to help incorporate microdosing into your daily routine. These tools include some of the lifestyle hacks described in "The Four Pillars (aka Four Food Groups) of Mental Health" on page 40, which are non-pharmaceutical practices of the biopsychosocial model of health; these will try to get you to see alternative views or stimulate thoughts.

This section has two separate parts; the first is to help you think about the journey you are preparing to embark on with grounding and setting an intention. Here I will offer some ideas about including exercise, meditation practices, and music to add some fun and excitement to help you along your microdosing journey.

The second part of this section helps guide you to make incremental steps toward your goals. Week to week there are different themes and skills to help stimulate thought, feeling, and emotion. Each week also builds upon the previous week's progress.

Before we go any further, I will offer you the scales and assessments that I mentioned in the guidebook portion.

The Microdosing Mood Chart on page 179 can help to track your mood and how it coincides with your microdose amount. In addition, you can track other factors that can be associated with microdosing/mood such as sleep, anxiety, exercise, pain, and physical changes or sensations (e.g., nausea, appetite changes, feeling "cloudy," or GI disturbances). Tracking will help you to determine your individual dosing regimen as you build a relationship with the substances. You can come up with your individual tracking methods. Zero should be an average day, neither good, nor bad; +5 should be the best day you have ever had in all your life; and -5 should be the worst day possible. Remember, this is individualized to you, and the most important piece is to be consistent with your scoring.

THE MICRODOSING MOOD CHART

PAIN	EXERCISE	LIFE CHANGES	ANXIETY	SLEEP	MOOD												MEDICATION CHANGES	MEDICATION AMOUNT	MONTH/WEEKDAY
					LOW						INCREASED								
					-5	-4	-3	-2	-1	0	+1	+2	+3	+4	+5				

PANAS QUESTIONNAIRE

This scale consists of a number of words that describe different feelings and emotions. Reach each item and then list the number from the scale below next to each word. Indicate to what extent you feel this way right now, that is, at the present moment, *OR* indicate the extent you have felt this way over the past week.

1	2	3	4	5
VERY SLIGHTLY OR NOT AT ALL	A LITTLE	MODERATELY	QUITE A BIT	EXTREMELY

___**1.** Interested

___**2.** Distressed

___**3.** Excited

___**4.** Upset

___**5.** Strong

___**6.** Guilty

___**7.** Scared

___**8.** Hostile

___**9.** Enthusiastic

___**10.** Proud

___**11.** Irritable

___**12.** Alert

___**13.** Ashamed

___**14.** Inspired

___**15.** Nervous

___**16.** Determined

___**17.** Attentive

___**18.** Jittery

___**19.** Active

___**20.** Afraid

SCORING INSTRUCTIONS

POSITIVE AFFECT SCORE: Add the scores on items 1, 3, 5, 9, 10, 12, 14, 16, 17, and 19. Scores can range from 10–50, with higher scores representing higher levels of positive affect.

NEGATIVE AFFECT SCORE: Add the scores on items 2, 4, 6, 7, 8, 11, 13, 15, 18, and 20. Scores can range from 10–50, with lower scores representing lower levels of negative affect.

Now take the total number from the Positive Affect Score and subtract the total from the Negative Affect Score. This will give you your total PANAS Score. The higher the number, the more positive your mood is, and vice versa.

PHQ-8: SCREENING TOOL FOR DEPRESSION

The PHQ (Kroenke, Spitzer, and Williams 2001) is a patient health questionnaire, a quick diagnostic tool used by many healthcare providers to measure an individual's mood/symptoms. Over time, the goal is to reduce these numbers. When answering these questions, reflect on how often these symptoms have affected you in the past two weeks.

HOW OFTEN HAVE YOU BEEN BOTHERED BY ANY OF THE FOLLOWING PROBLEMS?	PHQ-8	NOT AT ALL 0-1 DAY	SEVERAL DAYS 2-6 DAYS	MORE THAN HALF THE DAYS 7-11 DAYS	NEARLY EVERY DAY 12-14 DAYS
1. Little interest or pleasure in doing things		0	1	2	3
2. Feeling down, depressed, or hopeless		0	1	2	3
3. Trouble falling or staying asleep, or sleeping too much		0	1	2	3
4. Feeling tired or having little energy		0	1	2	3
5. Poor appetite or overeating		0	1	2	3
6. Feeling bad about yourself— or that you are a failure or have let yourself or your family down		0	1	2	3
7. Trouble concentrating on things, such as reading the newspaper or watching television		0	1	2	3
8. Moving or speaking so slowly that other people could have noticed. Or the opposite— being so fidgety or restless that you have been moving around a lot more than usual.		0	1	2	3

GAD-7: SCREENING TOOL FOR GENERALIZED ANXIETY DISORDER

The GAD-7 is a standard scale that mental health clinicians use to track progress when prescribing medications for generalized anxiety (Spitzer, Kroenke, and Lowe 2006).

OVER THE LAST 2 WEEKS, HOW OFTEN HAVE YOU BEEN BOTHERED BY THE FOLLOWING PROBLEMS?	NOT AT ALL	SEVERAL DAYS	MORE THAN HALF THE DAYS	NEARLY EVERY DAY
1. Feelings nervous, anxious, or on edge	0	1	2	3
2. Not being able to stop or control worrying	0	1	2	3
3. Worrying too much about different things	0	1	2	3
4. Trouble relaxing	0	1	2	3
5. Being so restless that it is hard to sit still	0	1	2	3
6. Becoming easily annoyed or irritable	0	1	2	3
7. Feelings afraid, as if something awful might happen	0	1	2	3

Total Score_____ = Add Columns _____ + _____ + _____ +

If you check off <u>any</u> problems, how <u>difficult</u> have these problems made it for you to do your work, take care of things at home, or get along with other people?

NOT DIFFICULT AT ALL	SOMEWHAT DIFFICULT	VERY DIFFICULT	EXTREMELY DIFFICULT
☐	☐	☐	☐

NOTES:

Use this section to write personal notes to yourself, thoughts you hope to answer in the future, or space to write some of the results from your questionnaires (allowing you to see how your results have changed over time).

NOTES:

THE MICRODOSING GUIDEBOOK

NOTES:

THE MICRODOSING GUIDEBOOK

SETTING GOALS

SETTING A GOAL: Goals are results focused.

HOW TO FIND SUCCESS:

- Be extremely specific about what it is that you want.

- Be persistent with yourself (and hold yourself accountable).

- Place what you want to achieve up close and personal. Eat, sleep, and breathe it every day until it happens.

- Setting small, incremental goals help many reach a larger goal.

Remember—Goals should be both measurable and attainable.

Some examples of goals for microdosing may be to get off medications (antidepressants, pain medications, anxiety medications), stick to a workout routine, or something arbitrary such as to organize your home or office.

WHAT ARE YOUR MICRODOSING AND LIFE GOALS?

- Daily goals (e.g., eat healthy, walk for thirty minutes, get adequate sleep)

- Goals for the week (e.g., plan meals, keep within a budget, visit a friend)

- Goals for the month (e.g., pay bills on time, drink less, lose weight)

- Goals for six weeks (e.g., plan a vacation, learn a new skill, work out 3x/week)

- Goals for three months (e.g., learn another language, run a 5K, go camping)

- Goals for six months (e.g., enroll in school, do home improvements)

- Goals for the year (e.g., earn an advancement at work, move to a new city)

SETTING YOUR INTENTION

Setting an intention while you are doing a microdosing protocol is extremely important, as it will help you to feel more connected to your reason for wanting to microdose. When you are living with intention, it's much more likely that you'll reach all your goals. Having a clear intention, and always looking for ways to live it, is the key to manifesting everything that you hope to get out of this course.

Intentions are not something with an outcome, and there's no way to evaluate them. An intention is something that you have a desire to bring into your life—so it's more aligned with the way you want to live. With intentions, your heart takes the wheel, and it is driven by a purpose.

HOW TO FIGURE OUT YOUR MICRODOSING JOURNEY INTENTION:

1. What matters most to you in life?

2. What areas in your life would you like to grow into?

3. What thoughts do you have that are holding you back?

4. What are you holding on to that no longer serves you?

5. When do you feel the happiest/most blissful/full of joy?

6. What are you grateful for?

MY TEN MICRODOSING JOURNEY INTENTIONS:

1. _____

2. _____

3. _____

4. _____

5. _____

6. _____

7. _____

8. _____

9. _____

10. _____

EXAMPLES OF INTENTIONS ARE:

🌀 My intention is to find forgiveness for myself.

🌀 My intention is to find forgiveness for others.

🌀 My intention is to stop letting fear hold me back from what I want.

🌀 My intention is to be more vulnerable.

🌀 My intention is to practice patience.

🌀 My intention is to love others unconditionally.

🌀 My intention is to connect with others.

🌀 My intention is to put energy into supportive relationships.

🌀 My intention is to embrace change and surrender to the flow.

🌀 My intention is to grow spiritually.

🌀 My intention is to be open to success and abundance.

HOW TO BE SUCCESSFUL WITH YOUR INTENTION:

- Use positive words that make you feel good. Instead of: "My intention is to stop hanging out with people who drain me," try this instead: "My intention is to put energy into supportive relationships."

- Continue working on your intentions and change them up as you evolve.

- Break down your intentions into more manageable parts.

- Celebrate your wins, both big and small.

- In order for your intention to come to light, it must be something you truly believe in and want for yourself. If it's something someone else wants for you, it won't work. Don't let the opinions, doubts, or influences of others distract you from what it is that you want.

- Remind yourself that by keeping to your intention, you are having a positive impact on the world and all the people in it. That's a pretty powerful motivation!

- Don't get so busy with life that you forget to enjoy the process.

- Don't lie to yourself by saying things like you're not good enough or not smart enough. Remember the truth. As Stuart Smalley of *Saturday Night Live* says, "You are good enough. You are smart enough. And gosh darn it, people like you!"

- Be consistent. Take a few minutes every single day to set your intention for microdosing. Use a journal to write down your intentions and also include all thoughts and observations you experience.

NOTE AREA

WHAT ARE YOUR THOUGHTS THUS FAR? What are some things that you have found important? What are your observations? Do you have questions? Who can help you answer your questions?

_____

_____

_____

_____

_____

_____

_____

_____

_____

_____

_____

_____

_____

_____

_____

_____

SELF-CARE

Arguably, one of the easiest and most effective ways to improve one's mental health is to introduce sustainable self-care practices. Introducing self-care practices as part of your microdosing journey can help you to get the most out of your journey and solidify these practices into your everyday routine. Remember, self-care can be anything that helps you to take time to rest, relax, reflect, replenish your energy, and renew. You must place a priority on your own needs, goals, health, and accomplishments while taking time to nourish and nurture all of who you are.

PHYSICAL SELF-CARE PRACTICES: These are practices of self-care that help one achieve living a healthy lifestyle. Some ideas are eating healthy, drinking enough water, physical exertion, and taking time to rest. Additionally, this also includes surrounding yourself with a clean, uncluttered, and comfortable environment.

SUGGESTIONS:

- Start your day drinking a pint of water.
- Add green vegetables to each meal.
- Go for a walk.
- Do a HIIT (high-intensity interval training) workout.
- Take a yoga class.
- Practice movement meditation.
- Practice guided meditation or mindfulness exercises.
- Dance.

🌀 Surround yourself with positive energy.

🌀 Get adequate sleep (and practice good sleep hygiene).

🌀 Declutter and organize your home, office, and bedroom.

🌀 Journal, reflect, and set goals!!!

What are you currently doing for your physical self-care?

_____

_____

_____

_____

_____

_____

_____

What could you do to up your physical self-care game?

_____

_____

_____

_____

_____

_____

Set one goal for yourself regarding physical self-care. What is it? What do you need to do to achieve it? When do you want to achieve your goal?

_____

_____

_____

_____

_____

_____

_____

_____

_____

_____

EMOTIONAL SELF-CARE: Emotional self-care can be seen as setting clear boundaries around your time, energy, or emotions. Have clear communication with others. Say no to what isn't in alignment and say yes to what is. Give and receiving support, kindness, and love. Spend time with people who care about you and your well-being. Get back from a relationship what you put in. Emotional self-care doesn't only include friends and family members, it also includes professional relationships and one's place of employment.

What are you currently doing for your emotional self-care?

_____

_____

_____

_____

_____

What could you do to improve your emotional self-care?

_____

_____

_____

_____

_____

Think of one relationship that you could improve for your emotional self-care; what would that look like? What do you need to do to improve it?

_____

_____

_____

_____

_____

PSYCHOLOGICAL SELF-CARE: Psychological self-care is self-care that has to do with mental and behavioral well-being. These include our thoughts, emotions (and emotional response), mood, and their accompanying symptoms.

SUGGESTIONS:

- Put your attention on things that are in your control.
- Reflect on what's going on in your life.
- Do mindfulness exercises.
- Meditate.
- Work with a therapist or health coach.
- Spend time in nature.

What are you currently doing for your psychological self-care?

_____

_____

_____

_____

_____

What could you do to improve your psychological self-care?

_____

_____

_____

_____

_____

PERSONAL SELF-CARE MENU

HOW TO DO IT:

🌀 Write down a list of twenty-five things that you love to do, that bring you joy and make you feel good.

   ○ Be sure to choose activities that have varying time commitments, from a couple of minutes to many hours.

🌀 Each day choose at least one activity from your menu to do.

🌀 Need help? See our sample self-care menu below!

SELF-CARE MENU

1. Go for a walk.

2. Write a letter to a friend.

3. Take a bath.

4. Put on a favorite song and dance to it.

5. Listen to your favorite song with your eyes closed.

6. Call a friend or family member.

7. Color.

8. Doodle.

9. Watch an uplifting video.

10. Make a healthy snack.

11. Meditate.

12. Gaze at a lit candle.

13. Put your hands on your heart and take three deep breaths.

14. Drink a warm cup of tea/coffee/lemon H2O.

15. Look out the window.

16. Stretch.

17. Write in your journal.

18. Watch an uplifting movie or TV show.

19. Read a book.

20. Exercise.

21. Do some yoga.

22. Repeat affirmations.

23. Take a nap.

24. Get out in nature.

25. Straighten up a room in your home.

Now, make your own list!

PERSONAL SELF-CARE MENU:

1. _____

2. _____

3. _____

4. _____

5. _____

6. _____

7. _____

8. _____

9. _____

10. _____

11. _____

12. _____

13. _____

14. _____

15. _____

16. _____

17. _____

18. _____

19. _____

20. _____

21. _____

22. _____

23. _____

24. _____

25. _____

CREATE YOUR MICRODOSE MYCO-MIXTAPE

Shout-out to my friend Taraleigh Weathers (www.rockinglife .com), who graciously gave me permission to keep her awesome idea of incorporating music into one's microdosing journey. Music not only soothes the savage beast, it also can magically bring us back to a different time and place in our lives. The idea here is to help make those positive connections.

Most people connect music to memories. When listening to music, you can instantly be transported back to when you first heard a song or associated that song with a memorable occasion. The music can touch a part of your soul that almost nothing else can. It's magic, healing, transformative, and medicinal. Music can bring to light memories, evoke feelings, and give you inspiration in your life. Microdosing does that, too! Life is better with a soundtrack, so let's create one. Here's how:

SOME RULES TO FOLLOW:

🌀 Don't choose more than two songs by the same artist.

🌀 The songs don't have to have lyrics.

🌀 Not all songs have to evoke happy feelings, but they *must* evoke feelings.

🌀 Cover songs are OK.

🌀 Live and studio-recorded songs are both OK.

Create your own Microdose Myco-Mixtape. I created two paths to get your soundtrack out of you. Try one or both of them, using songs from either path to make your final soundtrack.

PATH 1: USING THE PAST TO CREATE YOUR MIXTAPE

Begin this exercise by heart storming (like brainstorming, but with your heart) for twelve positive moments in your life. Here are some suggestions:

- First time you realized that music was important to you
- A family vacation
- A road trip
- A personal achievement
- First concert
- First kiss
- Sleepovers with your friends
- Wedding day
- First date
- An amazing party you attended
- First day of school
- Last day of school
- Graduation
- First day on the job
- Quitting your job
- Birth of a child

YOUR TWELVE MOMENTS:

1.

2.

3. _____

4. _____

5. _____

6. _____

7. _____

8. _____

9. _____

10. _____

11. _____

12. _____

Next to each moment write a short and sweet description or a couple of keywords that describe how you felt during that big event. These will be your liner notes. Using those moments and the feelings attached to them, choose songs that evoke those same feelings. It can be the actual song you were listening to or not.

YOUR SONGS:

1. _____

2. _____

3. _____

4. _____

5. _____

6. _____

7. _____

8. _____

9. _____

10. _____

11. _____

12. _____

Now, look at the songs on your mixtape and arrange them in any order of your choosing.

YOUR MIXTAPE ORDER:

1. _____

2. _____

3. _____

4. _____

5. _____

6. _____

7. _____

8. _____

9. _____

10. _____

11. _____

12. _____

TITLE OF YOUR SOUNDTRACK:

_____

PATH 2: USING YOUR FEELINGS (REMEMBER, SAME RULES APPLY)

Begin this exercise by coming up with one song that matches each of the following:

🌀 Song 1: Your strutting song (aka a song that brings out your inner John Travolta in the opening scene of Saturday Night Fever)

🌀 Song 2: Your song that just speaks to your soul

🌀 Song 3: Your getting-pumped-up song

🌀 Song 4: Your happy song

🌀 Song 5: Your nostalgia song

🌀 Song 6: Your song that makes you dance

🌀 Song 7: Your chilling/relaxing/calm song

🌀 Song 8: Your sexy song

🌀 Song 9: The song you know every word to

🌀 Song 10: The song that reminds you of "that time" (whatever "that time" means to you)

🌀 Song 11: The song you turn up really loud on a long drive

🌀 Song 12: Your favorite song ever!!!

YOUR TWELVE SONGS:

1. _____

2. _____

3. _____

4. _____

5. _____

6. _____

7. _____

8. _____

9. _____

10. _____

11. _____

12. _____

Next to each song choice write a short and sweet description or a couple of keywords that describe how you feel when you hear those songs. These will be your liner notes.

Look at the songs on your soundtrack and arrange them in any order of your choosing.

YOUR SOUNDTRACK ORDER:

1.

2.

3.

4.

5.

6.

7.

8.

9.

10.

11.

12.

NOW, WHAT IS THE NAME OF THIS MIXTAPE?

CHOOSING YOUR MICRODOSING THEME SONG

Choose one song from your soundtrack that encompasses the way you want to feel during your microdosing journey (or path) so you can bring that into your life in big ways by the time you complete week 6. Chances are you don't feel that way right now.

Some things to consider:

🌀 If you want to bring in love, choose a song that makes you feel you have that love right now. If you want to inhabit the sense of being free, choose a song that makes you feel that way. If you want to feel open to the magic of the universe and all the abundance it offers, choose a song that makes you believe that it's possible. If you want to feel calm and at peace, pick a song that brings up those sensations. Whatever way you want to feel is right.

🌀 You must at least kind of like this song/enjoy listening to it because you are going to be listening to it daily.

🌀 If this song isn't currently on your soundtrack, you may add it as a bonus track.

YOUR SONG:

_____

GET TO KNOW YOUR SONG:

🌀 Week 1: Listen to your song. When it's over, close your eyes, place your hands on your heart, take three deep breaths feeling the feelings it evoked in all your cells, open your eyes, and journal about it for a few minutes.

- Week 2: Read the lyrics of the song out loud.

- Week 3: Move to your song. Dance, sit and sway, bop your head, walk, etc.

- Week 4: Repeat week one.

BONUS TRACKS:

- Design the cover of your soundtrack. Draw it. Paint it. Use magazine clippings.

- Create a Spotify playlist.

- Get a pair of headphones and listen to your playlist in its entirety.

Listen to one song a day.

- Get dressed up and go for a walk while listening to your soundtrack.

- Share your soundtrack with your friends and challenge them to make their own.

- Take a screenshot of the cover of your soundtrack (if you made one), take another screenshot of your Spotify playlist, and finally, share your playlist to your social media.

  - Tag @Entheonurse using the hashtag #lifeisbetterwithasoundtrack.

WEEK 1: SETTING YOUR INTENTION

SETTING THE STAGE FOR CHANGE

This first week is about setting intentions. Before proceeding with this part, you should read and review Chapter 3 "The Biopsychosocial Model of Health," especially the section "The Four Pillars (aka Four Food Groups) of Mental Health" on page 40, and Chapter 5, "When to Start Journaling." While you read it, think about what it says and what it says to you. Then come back here to take some time to reflect.

PHYSICAL HEALTH: Describe your current physical health.

Things to consider: What is going well for your health? What could be better?

_____

_____

_____

_____

_____

_____

_____

_____

_____

PSYCHOLOGICAL/MENTAL HEALTH: Describe your current mental health.

Things to consider: What is going well for your mental health? What could be better? What could you do to improve your overall mental health?

_____

_____

_____

_____

_____

_____

_____

_____

_____

SOCIALIZATION AND ENVIRONMENTAL HEALTH: Describe your current socialization/environmental health (e.g., family life, social life, school, work, hobbies, lifestyle, and interactions with nature).

Things to consider: What is going well for you and how you interact with others and the world around you? Do you have a healthy balance? What could be better? What could you do to improve how you interact with others?

_____

_____

_____

_____

_____

_____

_____

_____

PUTTING IT ALL TOGETHER

Do you feel that you have a healthy balance between those three components of the biopsychosocial model (physical, mental, social health)?

Things to consider: What part do you feel you identify with the most? The least? Why?

_____

_____

_____

_____

_____

_____

What would having a healthy balance of those parts look like for you?

_____

_____

_____

_____

_____

_____

_____

_____

_____

SETTING INTENTION: Now that you have taken time to think about what makes up who you are and the areas in your life for personal growth, let's look at how to get there. You may have some ideas from your answers about yourself and your physical, mental, and social health.

In this first week of your *Microdosing Guidebook* program, the goal is to set your intention for the program. This may seem like a difficult goal at first, but think back and reflect on what made you want to participate in the program in the first place.

What did you hope to learn or change about yourself, and what did you feel that this journey could help you achieve? Why did you feel this program could help you? Look deeply within. No one needs to know these answers but you.

Take a moment to reflect on these questions and describe your intention.

_____

_____

_____

_____

_____

WEEK 2: GETTING TO KNOW YOUR FUN-GUYS (OR GALS, OR GENDER NONCONFORMING)

Despite this being the second week of the microdosing journey, this is when you are scheduled to start your microdosing. The first week we started with pre-integration, getting to know yourself, and setting your intention for your *Microdosing Guidebook*. Now you want to get to know your fungi and start to be mindful of how the microdose is affecting you.

Things to consider: This week you are starting your protocol, which means it is important to practice mindfulness and self-awareness so you can be aware of how the medicine is affecting you. Are you having new sensations? Are they comfortable? Uncomfortable? Is it tolerable?

If you are not noticing changes, that's OK... That's why we are doing this.

PHYSICALLY: How are your microdoses affecting you physically? Think about the following questions: the day before starting (your baseline), dosing day, and the days after.

Did the microdose make you feel physically uncomfortable? How so?

_____

_____

_____

_____

MENTALLY: How is your microdose affecting you mentally? Think about the following questions: the day before starting (your baseline), dosing day, and the days after.

Did the microdose make you feel mentally uncomfortable? How so?

_____

_____

_____

_____

_____

_____

_____

_____

_____

_____

_____

SOCIALIZATION AND ENVIRONMENTAL HEALTH: How is your microdose affecting you socially? Think about the following questions: the day before starting (your baseline), dosing day, and the days after.

Did the microdose make you feel socially uncomfortable or uncomfortable around others? How so?

_____

_____

_____

_____

_____

_____

_____

_____

_____

_____

SPIRITUALLY: How is your microdose affecting you spiritually? Think about the following questions: the day before starting (your baseline), dosing day, and the days after.

Did the microdose make you feel closer to people, other living things, or nature? How so?

_____

_____

_____

_____

_____

_____

_____

_____

_____

_____

End-of-the-Week Evaluation: Take a moment to reflect on your week. Overall, how do you feel your program is going? Do you feel like you are making personal growth?

How are you progressing with your intention?

_____

_____

_____

_____

_____

_____

_____

_____

_____

Next week's theme is "Spreading Your Mycelium Network of Self"

Take this space to write something encouraging to yourself this week and something you hope to learn about next week.

WEEK 3: SPREADING YOUR MYCELIUM NETWORK OF SELF

The reported effects of psychedelics include a sense of increased connection with nature and the mystical qualities of internal/external unity. Now, in your third week of the microdosing journey, the plan is to start spreading yourself and affecting your environment around you. As we learned in the biopsychosocial model of health, we know how all living things are interconnected and share energy.

Take these thoughts into the third week of this journey. As you have started to dial into finding your sweet spot for dosing, you want to start to make small, subtle changes to improve your life.

Things to Consider: This third week you are in the second week of your protocol, which means it is important to practice mindfulness and self-awareness of your own personal growth. This week you are looking at your connection to others around you (e.g., family, friends, coworkers, anyone around you) and how you interact with them. As you dial into finding your sweet spot for dosing, you want to start to make small, subtle changes to improve your life.

BACKGROUND: Have you ever heard the Japanese term *shinrin-yoku*? Translated, *shinrin* means "forest" and *yoku* means "bath," or immersing oneself in the forest and soaking in the atmosphere through the senses. Research has shown this to decrease cortisol levels and lower pulse, blood pressure, and other biological markers for stress; ultimately, it is good for your physical and mental health.

"...to walk in the forest and observe your thoughts."

—Hofmann (Passie 2019, 24) on using low-dose LSD

To Do: Challenge yourself, like Hofmann, to mindfully walk for at least thirty minutes in nature once this week (no headphones). Observe your surroundings and senses. What did you see? Smell? Taste? Hear? Feel? Notice anything giving off energy during the walk? If so, describe it. Do you feel a connection with the world around you? How so? Let your network grow around you.

Is there anything you can do to improve your connection to the world around you? What would it take for you to make those improvements? If you're stumped, ask a trusted friend or family member: What can you do?

_____

_____

_____

_____

_____

_____

_____

_____

_____

PHYSICAL EFFECTS: Reflect on the perceived effects of the dosing. Have you noticed any effects? How are you feeling?

Any uncomfortable feelings? Are they tolerable? Too much? Too little?

_____

_____

_____

_____

_____

_____

_____

_____

PSYCHOSOCIAL: How are your microdoses affecting your psychosocial needs? Think about this throughout the protocol cycle.

Have you felt an increased sense of connection with others (e.g., friends, family, coworkers, another friend who is microdosing with you, other living things, nature, what you enjoy doing)? How so?

WEEK 4: HOW MUSHROOM DO YOU HAVE TO GROW?

Now in your fourth week of the microdosing journey, the plan is to start making larger changes (with the help of your microdosing protocol). Take advantage of how your medicine changes the way you think and how you see the world around you. The medicine can help you to see new pathways around challenges—use that to make life changes.

Things to Consider: In this fourth week of dosing, I hope you are starting to notice some changes. These changes are hopefully helping you to grow closer to your optimal self and closer to your intentions. Growth can be uncomfortable— physically, emotionally, socially, or spiritually—but ask yourself if that growth is uncomfortable or if you are being challenged. Sometimes we may need to ask ourselves "What is the consequence of not changing or not growing?" Not changing and not growing can have untoward effects or may be self-destructive.

Change can be tough, that's why we often avoid change or may be slow to make changes. So, I ask you: How mushroom do you have to make changes or how mushroom do you have to grow? Like mushrooms, humans have more connections than what appears at the surface. We, too, have a mycelium network connecting all of us, and this network may help us grow.

BACKGROUND: Sometimes we need help to grow, change, and progress forward; this is where your mycelium network can help you to grow forth. Our social circle (e.g., friends, family, coworkers) is sometimes the best resource to help us to reach our goals and achieve our intention. These people can help us see things differently or encourage us when growth may appear challenging.

The COVID era taught us that we need to distance ourselves physically and socially in order to protect ourselves and those around us. The process of isolation has its own drawbacks and consequences as well. Loneliness can lead to poorer outcomes in both physical and mental health. Sarvada Chandra Tiwari (2013) writes about how there are three types of loneliness: situational, developmental, and internal.

🌀 Situational loneliness is influenced by socioeconomic status and the culture we live in. One may argue we are all dealing with situational loneliness on some level due to social isolation during COVID, limiting contact and interactions in the community, and meeting with one another over the computer instead of face-to-face.

🌀 Developmental loneliness is influenced by our desire to relate to one another or for intimacy. Developmental loneliness can also be influenced by one's sense that they are now growing or reaching personal milestones at the same rate as others or by societal standards. We should remember that personal development, physical factors, and psychiatric issues also influence reaching one's developmental milestones.

🌀 Internal loneliness is influenced by how one feels. Being alone does not always equate to a sense of isolation; it is the perception of being alone. Having low self-esteem or feeling a sense of inadequacy or low self-worth also can contribute to feeling lonely.

Building a strong support system, maintaining strong self-care practices, and feeling a connection or a part of something increases our self-worth, which in turn decreases our sense of loneliness. This support system can also help us through the challenges and discomfort of personal change and self-growth.

To Do: Reaching out and improving contact with others will help you to grow personally. It may not be you who is truly in need of reaching out; it might be the other person who needs someone to reach out to them. Take some time to think about who you should reach out to.

Name three people who may benefit from talking with you. Why?

_____

_____

_____

_____

_____

Name three people who you may benefit talking with. Why?

_____

_____

_____

_____

_____

Now challenge yourself to contact one person from each of these lists. Who will you contact? What will you talk about?

_____

_____

_____

_____

_____

_____

_____

In the next week, what will you do to help you achieve your intention for this program? Can anyone that you have named in the previous questions help you to achieve your goals or intentions? Will you ask them? Why or why not?

_____

_____

_____

_____

_____

_____

_____

_____

What do you feel is your greatest challenge that is preventing you from growing? What do you think you may be able to do to change that?

_____

_____

_____

_____

_____

_____

_____

_____

Are there any habits you have learned (or are now instilling) that are helping you grow?

_____

_____

_____

_____

_____

_____

How do you feel about your microdosing regimen? Do you feel it has helped you grow? Have you been experiencing any intolerable side effects? Do you feel like you have been benefiting?

_____

_____

_____

_____

_____

_____

_____

_____

WEEK 5: NOT TRIPPIN', STRAIGHT UP LIVIN'

Now in your fifth week of the microdosing journey, the plan is to start making these newfound thoughts, feelings, and emotions into a long-term lifestyle. This journey is not intended to be like a six-week restricted diet, it is a six-week overhaul to help you reach your optimal self. It's a time to live your best life with the help of the protocol and the work you have put into the workbook.

Things to Consider: By this point in the program, you should be starting to get an idea of how the microdosing affects you physically, mentally, and emotionally. Ask yourself (and reflect over your journals) if what you feel is working or not working. Do you feel any benefits on dosing days and the day after? If you haven't noticed anything, have you increased your dosage? Remember, a microdose of psilocybin is one-tenth of a normal high dose (which for some may be between 0.3 grams to 0.5 grams).

Besides the microdosing protocols, what other changes have you incorporated into your life during this program? Have you felt an increased sense of creativity? Connection? Increased energy? Better health habits?

This week is about understanding how to incorporate changes into living your life. Take a moment to reflect on the personal growth you may have experienced in this program.

What are some changes you plan to implement? Remember this is a new start for a new you... Time for some straight-up livin'.

_____

_____

_____

_____

_____

_____

_____

_____

Setting goals for yourself is a great way to keep your focus forward. What is one goal for you to accomplish this week?

_____

_____

_____

What is one goal for the month?

_____

_____

_____

What is one goal for six months from now?

_____

What is one goal to accomplish before the end of the year?

_____

_____

_____

What is one goal to accomplish in five years?

_____

_____

_____

What is one goal to accomplish in ten years?

_____

_____

_____

Who can help you to accomplish those goals?

_____

_____

_____

WEEK 6: INTEGRATION. WHAT'S NEXT?

In this final week of *The Microdosing Guidebook* program, we hope you have been able to find your sweet spot for your personal microdose. You have had a few weeks of trial-and-error dosages to see what has been beneficial or tolerable (if you have experienced side effects), and have had time to reflect what it does for your body.

During this time we have reviewed ways to also improve your life, such as relaxation techniques, exercise, mindfulness techniques, journaling, and exploring your "mycelium" network. What is going to happen next? Take time to think about where you started and how far you have come. Have you grown? Have you met your intention? You have made changes, and are they sustainable? Have you found the sweet spot for dosing? Do you plan to continue?

Now that you have a better idea of what your sweet spot is, ask yourself if taking it every four days is too much time in between? Is it too short, and might you benefit from once-a-week dosing? Only you know that. Review your journal entries and see what you need.

Things to Consider: The improvements you have made could be because of the microdosing regimen, or because time has passed, or because of the other skills you have learned... all of this could be because of a placebo effect. Whatever the case, I truly hope you have gained insight into yourself, your place in the world, and the world around you.

You can continue to microdose and follow your regimen... you could stop and return when you feel you need it. Next time you will be ready and know what dosage would be best for you.

To Do: Find two dates about six months from now and a year from now. Mark them in your calendar. On those dates, come back to your workbook and journal. Review what you have gained. Ask yourself the same questions you answered in this workbook. See where you stand and if answers have changed.

What has been your biggest win or achievement in the previous six weeks? (Was it your original intention? Was it something bigger?)

_____

_____

_____

_____

_____

What is something you have done that you feel you want to continue (e.g., taking walks in nature regularly, reaching out to others more, breathing exercises, microdosing, yoga, journaling...)?

_____

_____

_____

_____

_____

What have you learned or gained the most from this program?

_____

_____

_____

_____

_____

What are your plans now that this program has concluded?

_____

_____

_____

_____

_____

Link to a study that is looking at microdosing and self-blinding effects:

https://selfblinding-microdose.org/sign-up

MY JOURNEY AND THE CATCH-22 OF PSYCHEDELIC WRITING

I know it is unconventional, but I consciously decided to tell my story at the end of the book. While I feel it is important to tell my story in order to help decrease the stigma associated with these sacred medicines, I also understand that had I self-disclosed my personal relationship with these substances earlier, I might affect the reader's perception of the material I presented. Research has that when writers self-disclose their psychedelic use, people's perception of their work and the writer's integrity is affected negatively. So here lies the catch-22 and why I decided to tell this at the end.

Early in my adult life, all I really knew about psychedelic substances was that they could be a fun escape from reality, using them to have fun with friends on a hike in nature or sitting on the bank of a river running through the middle of a college town, staring off into the distance (or looking deeply inward) while listening to Phish. They were truly for recreational purposes. Sure, I had heard about how they were used in the '50s and '60s, and they were responsible for tie-dye, Woodstock, and changing the Beatles from the clean-cut look that they had when they first came from England to the *Magical Mystery Tour* group of hippies that changed music forever, but their medicinal use was often presented as dismissive. This view was also clouded by visions of how drugs will ruin our brains like an egg smashing into a frying pan.

Fast-forward to early spring 2018. Up to this point, all my encounters with psychedelics had been either strictly recreational or through patients who presented to the hospital in the midst of a "bad trip" or similar negative drug experience. On that fateful day, I had a patient who came into my emergency department presenting as manic and psychotic, but what was interesting was he was in his late fifties or early sixties and didn't have any known psychiatric history. His treatment was pretty routine, and once stabilized, he sheepishly admitted that he had tried to self-medicate with psilocybin mushrooms; the exact strain is known as "Penis Envy."

Instantly, I was intrigued and thirsting to learn more. Honestly, this is a case where you need to be mindful of what you search for on the internet, but once I added the term "psychiatric," my results were more suitable for what I was looking for. I started to learn about Dr. Steven Pollock's research and beliefs in mushrooms as medicine (1975), and his eventual murder (Morris 2013). I started to request old publications on psychedelic medicines and read them all. The school's librarian must have hated me, as I am sure most of the requests were archived on microfiche. I questioned why this information wasn't better known. Then, a few months later, Michael Pollan's *How to Change Your Mind* (2018) was released, and that all changed. People were starting to know, and they weren't just mental health professionals.

For grad school that fall, I had to present an educational project for one of my classes. I discussed wanting to present on psychedelic research, its history, and efficacy. While my professor seemed skeptical, she was supportive, and it was well received by both the class and the group at work I presented to as required by the class. My presentation was made to mental health professionals, which included psychiatrists, nurses, social workers, and technicians. From that point, I was known as the psychedelic guy, but hey, there could be worse things, right?

The following spring, in 2019, I figured what the hell, and I submitted an abstract to the American Psychiatric Nurses Association for their national conference. Not thinking much about it, I was convinced that there was no way in hell they would pick me or my topic. It was too controversial and nonconventional. I kind of forgot about it, to be honest. Then, a few weeks later, I checked my email and my jaw dropped. I was breathless. I was confused. I was in shock. I was chosen as a podium presenter and was going to be placed in the psychopharmacology track, the highest attended due to contact hours needed for credentialing for advanced practice nurses (APRNs). This was the first time they had ever had a presentation on psychedelic substances.

During the writing and refining process, I had the epiphany that I needed to not miss anything, and I needed to search deeply to capture it all. There was only one logistical way to achieve this. I needed guidance from the mushroom. Like I said earlier, we were acquainted, but now I was doing it for a purpose. A few weeks later, after I acquired my guide, I decided that I needed to follow the encouragement of Albert Hofmann and be surrounded by nature. I wanted to be somewhere safe, where I knew I could be alone to do my work,[7] so I decided on a lovely island that is only accessible by a five-minute boat ride across the river.

It was a hot and sunny day in Maine. I packed up hiking supplies in my boat, mixed up a bottle of orange juice with a few grams of mycological medicine to soak for a lemon tek, and set off across the river. Once I landed, I made sure everything was prepared, I messaged friends to let them know what I was doing and where I was, drank my orange juice, and set off across the island. I know this place very well and felt comfortable there. My set and setting were on point. I brought snacks, water, tick repellent, and a hammock. I didn't know exactly what my plan would be, but I had about five miles to the other end of the island and had faith in my mycological co-pilot.

During my hike I experienced mysticism, awe, and wonder; shock; timelessness; oneness with nature; and ineffability. I stopped to watch deer, ducks, and bald eagles. I was amazed and, serendipitously, the hike ended as I neared the far side of the island. I was able to take my time hiking back to enjoy

---

7. For the record, I do not encourage this behavior. But if you decide to do so, be safe. Just like if you were to go solo hiking, have a plan, make others aware of the plan, and have communication available.

the comedown and try to piece together all that I took in. Some of the largest takeaways from that day for me were that I needed to share this amazing medicine with others. There was something more to it and I needed to be a part of the process. In order to honor that day effectively, the medicine told me that I need to trust it, follow it, and have faith in the path it would lead me. I know this may sound crazy to many people, and I don't like or use that term, but if you have had a psychedelic experience, you may know what I am talking about.

Lastly, I learned that in order to bring the message forward, I needed to have a name to define or distinguish myself from others. Then it hit me. I am a nurse, and thanks to my undergrad program, I was well versed in holistic nursing and the caring model of Jean Watson. What is holistic nursing? Caring a treatment of the whole person, not just a diagnosis or disorder. But, how do psychedelics fit into that? Then it hit me. Unlike the standard medical model that healthcare follows and the pharmaceutical approaches to treatment, psychedelics have the unique ability to treat from the inside. Individuals choosing to use psychedelic medicines are doing so to treat themselves, even if there is nothing pathologically wrong. One may use psychedelic substances to help achieve a level of wholeness or better understand themselves physically, spiritually, emotionally, or socially. That was when I understood I needed to use the term "EntheoNurse." An entheogen is a plant (including fungi), drug, or medicine that helps to invoke a spiritual experience. Entheogen is a neologism that comes from the Greek roots of en (within)- theo (divine)- and gen (creates), which translates to "creating the divine within."

REFERENCES

American Psychiatric Association. *Diagnostic and Statistical Manual of Mental Disorders (DSM–5), Fifth Edition.* Washington, DC: American Psychiatric Association Publishing, 2013.

Anderson, Thomas, Rotem Petranker, Adam Christopher, Daniel Rosenbaum, Cory Weissman, Le-Anh Dinh-Williams, Katrina Hui, Emma Hapke, and Norman A. S. Farb. "Microdosing Psychedelics: Personality, Mental Health, and Creativity Differences in Microdosers." *Psychopharmacology* 236, no. 2 (2019): 731–740. https://doi.org/10.1007/s00213-018-5106-2.

Anderson, Thomas, Rotem Petranker, Adam Christopher, Daniel Rosenbaum, Cory Weissman, Le-Anh Dinh-Williams, Katrina Hui, and Emma Hapke. "Psychedelic Microdosing Benefits and Challenges: An Empirical Codebook." *Harm Reduction Journal* 16, no. 43 (2019). https://doi.org/10.1186/s12954-019-0308-4.

Andersson, Martin, Mari Persson, and Anette Kjellgren. "Psychoactive Substances As a Last Resort—A Qualitative Study of Self-treatment of Migraine and Cluster Headaches." *Harm Reduction Journal* 14, no. 60 (2017). https://doi.org/10.1186/s12954-017-0186-6.

Anthony, J., A. Winstock, A., J. Ferris, J., and D. Nutt. "Improved Colour Blindness Symptoms Associated with Recreational Psychedelic Use: Results from the Global Drug Survey 2017." Drug Science, Policy and Law 6 (2020). https://doi.org/10.1177/2050324520942345.

Augsberger. Letter to Hanscarl Leuner, December 22, 1959.

Baer, Jack. "Dana White Says UFC Looking into Research on Microdosing Psychedelics to Combat Brain Trauma." Yahoo!Sports. January 13, 2021. https://sports.yahoo.com/dana-white-ufc-microdosing-psychedelics-fighters-brain-injuries-spencer-fisher-060126364.html.

Bauer, Barbara E. "Chemical Composition Variability in Magic Mushrooms." *Psychedelic Science Review*. March 4, 2019. https://psychedelicreview.com/chemical-composition-variability-in-magic-mushrooms.

Beakley B. D., A. M. Kaye, A. D. Kaye. "Tramadol, Pharmacology, Side Effects, and Serotonin Syndrome: A Review." *Pain Physician.* 2015;18:395–400.

Beecher, Henry K. "The Powerful Placebo." *Journal of the American Medical Association* 159, no. 17 (1955): 1602–1606. https://doi.org/10.1001/jama.1955.02960340022006.

Bender, Lauretta, D. V. Sika Sankar, Samuel Irwin, and Jose Egozcue. "Chromosome Damage Not Found in Leukocytes of Children Treated with LSD-25. *Science* 159, no. 3816 (1968): 749. https://doi.org/10.1126/science.159.3816.749.

Bershad, Anya K., Katrin H. Preller, Royce Lee, Sarah Keedy, Jamie Wren-Jarvis, Michael P. Bremmer, and Harriet de Wit. "Preliminary Report on the Effects of a Low Dose of LSD on Resting-State Amygdala Functional Connectivity.

Biological Psychiatry: Cognitive Neuroscience and Neuroimaging 5, no. 4 (2020): 461–467. https://doi.org/10.1016/j.bpsc.2019.12.007.

Bershad, Anya K., Scott T. Schepers, Michael P. Bremmer, Royce Lee, and Harriet de Wit. "Acute Subjective and Behavioral Effects of Microdoses of Lysergic Acid Diethylamide in Healthy Human Volunteers." *Biological Psychiatry* 86, no. 10 (2019): 792–800. https://doi.org/10.1016/j.biopsych.2019.05.019.

Blewett, D. B. and N. Chewlos. *Handbook for the Therapeutic Use of LSD: Individual and Group Procedures*, 1959. PDF. https://maps.org/research-archive/ritesofpassage/lsdhandbook.pdf.

Bonson, Katherine R. and D. L. Murphy. "Alterations in Responses to LSD in Humans Associated with Chronic Administration of Tricyclic Antidepressants, Monoamine Oxidase Inhibitors or Lithium." *Behavioral Brain Research* 73, no. 1–2 (1996): 229–33. https://doi.org/10.1016/0166-4328(96)00102-7.

Bonson, Katherine R., Joshua W. Buckholtz, and Dennis L. Murphy. "Chronic Administration of Serotonergic Antidepressants Attenuates the Subjective Effects of LSD in Humans." *Neuropsychopharmacology* 14 (1996): 425–436. https://doi.org/10.1016/0893-133X(95)00145-4.

Bornemann, Joel. "The Viability of Microdosing Psychedelics as a Strategy to Enhance Cognition and Well-Being—An Early Review." *Journal of Psychoactive Drugs* 52, no. 4 (2020): 300–308. https://doi.org/10.1080/02791072.2020.1761573.

Brandrup, E., and T. Vanggaard. "LSD Treatment in a Severe Case of Compulsive Neurosis." *Acta Psychiatrica Scandinavica* 55, no. 2, (1977): 127. https://doi.org/10.1111/j.1600-0447.1977.tb00149.x.

Brandt, Simon D., Pierce V. Kavanagh, Folker Westphal, Alexander Stratford, Simon P. Elliott, Khoa Hoang, Jason Wallach, and Adam L. Halberstadt. "Return of The Lysergamides. Part I: Analytical and Behavioural Characterization of 1-Propionyl-D-Lysergic Acid Diethylamide (1P-LSD)." *Drug Testing and Analysis* 8, no. 9 (2016): 891–902. https://doi.org/10.1002/dta.1884.

Brown, Walter A. "Placebo as a Treatment for Depression." *Neuropsychopharmacology* 10, no. 4 (1994): 265–269. https://doi.org/10.1038/npp.1994.53.

Brown, Walter. A. *The Placebo Effect in Clinical Practice.* Oxford: Oxford University Press, 2012.

Buchborn, Tobias, Gisela Grecksch, D. C. Dieterich. "Tolerance to Lysergic Acid Diethylamide: Overview, Correlates, and Clinical Implications." In *Neuropathology of Drug Addictions and Substance Misuse, Volume 2: Stimulants, Club and Dissociative Drugs, Hallucinogens, Steroids, Inhalants and International Aspects.* New York: Academic Press, 846–858, 2016.

Buchborn, Tobias, Helmut Schröder, Volker Höllt, and Gisela Grecksch. "Repeated Lysergic Acid Diethylamide in an Animal Model of Depression: Normalisation of Learning Behaviour and Hippocampal Serotonin 5-HT2 Signalling." *Journal of Psychopharmacology* 28, no. 6 (2014): 545–552. https://doi.org/10.1177/0269881114531666.

Buller, Kyle and Joe Moore. "Breaking Convention Series: Dr. Torsten Passie–The Science of Microdosing Psychedelics." *Psychedelics Today*. July 30, 2019. Podcast. https://psychedelicstoday.com/2019/07/30/breaking -convention-series-dr-torsten-passie-the-science-of -microdosing-psychedelics.

Buller, Kyle and Joe Moore. "PT 245: Robin Carhart-Harris– Psychedelics, Entropy, and Plasticity." *Psychedelics Today*. Podcast. May 25, 2021. https://psychedelicstoday. com/2021/05/25/pt245-robin-carhart-harris-psychedelics -entropy-and-plasticity.

Buller, Kyle and Joe Moore. "PT224: Dr. Dan Engle— The Concussion Repair Manual." *Psychedelics Today*. Podcast. December 19, 2020. https://psychedelicstoday. com/2020/12/29/pt224-dr-dan-engle-the-concussion-repair -manual.

Buller, Kyle and Joe Moore. "PTSD 50: Microdosing and the Placebo Effect, with Balázs Szigeti and David Erritzoe." *Psychedelics Today*. Podcast. March 12, 2021. https:// psychedelicstoday.com/2021/03/12/ptsf50-microdosing-and -the-placebo-effect-with-balazs-szigeti-and-david-erritzoe.

Burns, David D. *The Feeling Good Handbook*. New York: Plume, 1990.

Callaway, J. C. "Set, Setting, and Dose." In *Handbook of Medical Hallucinogens*, edited by Charles S. Grob and Jim Grisby, 347–362. New York: Guilford Press, 2021.

Cameron, Lindsay P., Angela Nazarian, and David E. Olson. "Psychedelic Microdosing: Prevalence and Subjective Effects." *Journal of Psychoactive Drugs* 52, no. 2 (2020): 113–122. https://doi.org/10.1080/02791072.2020.1718250.

Cameron, Lindsay P., Charlie J. Benson, Brian C. DeFelice, Oliver Fioehn, and David E. Olson. "Chronic, Intermittent Microdoses of the Psychedelic *N,N*-Dimethyltryptamine (DMT) Produce Positive Effects on Mood and Anxiety in Rodents." *ACS Chemical Neuroscience* 10, no. 7 (2019):3261–3270. https://doi.org/10.1021/acschemneuro.8b00692.

Carbonaro, Theresa M., Matthew P. Bradstreet, Frederick S. Barrett, Katherine A. MacLean, Robert Jesse, Matthew W. Johnson, and Roland R. Griffiths. "Survey Study of Challenging Experiences After Ingesting Psilocybin Mushrooms: Acute and Enduring Positive and Negative Consequences." *Journal of Psychopharmacology (Oxford)* 30, no. 12 (2016): 1268–1278. https://doi .org/10.1177/0269881116662634.

Carhart-Harris, Robin L. and David J. Nutt. "Serotonin and Brain Function: A Tale of Two Receptors." *Journal of Psychopharmacology (Oxford)* 31, no. 9 (2017): 1091–1120. https://doi.org/10.1177/0269881117725915.

Carhart-Harris, Robin L., David Erritzoe, Tim Williams, James M. Stone, Laurence J. Reed, Alessanddro Colasanti, Robin J. Tyacke, et al. "Neural Correlates of the Psychedelic State as Determined by fMRI Studies with Psilocybin." *Proceedings of the National Academy of Sciences* 109, no. 6 (2012): 2138–2143. https://doi.org/10.1073/pnas.1119598109.

Carhart-Harris, Robin, Bruna Gribaldi, Rosalind Watts, Michelle Baker-Jones, Ashleigh Murphy-Beiner, Roberta Murphy, Jonny Martell, Allan Bleminsg, David Erritzoe, and David J. Nutt. "Trial of Psilocybin Versus Escitalopram for Depression." *The New England Journal of Medicine* 384, no.

15 (2021): 1402–1411. https://doi.org/10.1056/NEJMoa 2032994.

Castellanos, Joel P., Chris Woolley, Kelly Amanda Bruno, Fadel Zeidan, Adam Halberstadt, and Timothy Furnish. "Chronic Pain and Psychedelics: A Review and Proposed Mechanism of Action." *Regional Anesthesia and Pain Medicine* 45, no. 7 (2020): 486–494. http://dx.doi.org/10.1136/rapm-2020 -101273.

Catlow, Briony J., Shijie Song, Daniel A. Paredes, Cheryl L. Kirstein, and Juan Sanchez-Ramos. "Effects of Psilocybin on Hippocampal Neurogenesis and Extinction of Trace Fear Conditioning." *Experimental Brain Research* 228, no.4 (2013): 481–491. https://doi.org/10.1007/s00221-013-3579-0.

Charnay, Yves and Lucienne Leger. "Brain Serotonergic Circuitries." *Dialogues in Clinical Neuroscience* 12, no. 4 (2010): 471–487. https://doi.org/10.31887/DCNS.2010.12.4 /ycharnay.

Charron, Alexandra, Cynthia El Hage, Alice Servonnet, and Anne-Noel Samaha. "5-HT2 Receptors Modulate the Expression of Antipsychotic-Induced Dopamine Supersensitivity." *European Neuropsychopharmacology* 25, no. 12 (2015): 2381–2393. https://doi.org/10.1016/j.euro neuro.2015.10.002.

Chouinard, Guy, Anne-Noel Samaha, Virginie-Anne Chouinard, Charles-Siegfried Peretty, Nobuhisa Kanahara, Masayuki Takase, and Masaomi Iyo. "Antipsychotic-Induced Dopamine Supersensitivity Psychosis: Pharmacology, Criteria, and Therapy." *Psychotherapy and Psychosomatics* 86, no. 4 (2017): 189–219. https://doi.org/10.1159/000 477313.

Cipriani, Andrea, Toshi A. Furukawa, Georgia Salanti, Anna Chaimani, Lauren Z. Atkinson, Yusuke Ogawa, Stefan Leucht, et al. "Comparative Efficacy and Acceptability of 21 Antidepressant Drugs for the Acute Treatment of Adults with Major Depressive Disorder: A Systematic Review and Network Meta-Analysis." *The Lancet* 391, no. 10128 (2018): 1357–1366. https://doi.org/10.1016/s0140-6736(17)32802-7.

Clark, Carey S. *Cannabis: A Handbook for Nurses*. Philadelphia: Lippincott, 2021.

Cohen, Sidney. "Lysergic Acid Diethylamide: Side Effects and Complications". *The Journal of Nervous and Mental Disease* 130, no. 30 (1960): 30–40. https://doi.org/10.1097/00005053 -196001000-00005.

Cuijpers, Pim, Marit Sijbrandij, Sander L. Koole, Gerhard Andersson, Aartjan T. Beekman, and Charles F. Reynolds III. "Adding Psychotherapy to Antidepressant Medication in Depression and Anxiety Disorders: A Meta-Analysis." *World Psychiatry* 13, no. 1 (2014): 56–67. https://doi.org/10.1002 /wps.20089.

Delgado, Pedro L. and Francisco A. Moreno. "Hallucinogens, Serotonin and Obsessive-Compulsive Disorder." *Journal of Psychoactive Drugs* 30, no. 4 (2011): 359–366. https://doi.org /10.1080/02791072.1998.10399711.

Dinan, Timothy G., and John F. Cryan. "Brain-Gut-Microbiota Axis and Mental Health." *Psychosomatic Medicine* 79, no. 8 (2017): 920–926. https://doi.org/10.1097/PSY .0000000000000519.

Dinan, Timothy G., and John F. Cryan. "The Impact of Gut Microbiota on Brain and Behaviour: Implications for Psychiatry." *Current Opinion in Clinical Nutrition and*

Metabolic Care 18, no. 6 (2015): 552–8. https://doi.org/10
.1097/MCO.0000000000000221.

Dolder, Patrick C., Yasmin Schmid, Andrea E. Steuer, Thomas
Kraemer, Katharina M. Rentsch, Felix Hammann, and Matthias E. Liechti. "Pharmacokinetics and Pharmacodynamics
of Lysergic Acid Diethylamide in Healthy Subjects." *Clinical
Pharmacokinetics* 56, no. 10 (2017): 1219–1230. https://doi
.org/10.1007/s40262-017-0513-9.

Dressler, Hannah M., Stephen J. Bright, and Vince Polito.
"Exploring the Relationship Between Microdosing,
Personality and Emotional Insight: A Prospective Study."
Journal of Psychedelic Studies 5, no. 1 (2021): 9–16. https://
doi.org/10.1556/2054.2021.00157.

Elyse, Bailey. "Long-Term Effects of Microdosing
Psychedelics." *Double Blind.* Last updated May 26, 2021.
https://doubleblindmag.com/long-term-effects-of
-microdosing-psychedelics.

Erritzoe, D., L. Roseman, M. M. Nour, K. MacLean, M. Kaelen,
D. J. Nutt, and R. L. Carhart-Harris. "Effects of Psilocybin
Therapy on Personality Structure." *Acta Psychiatrica
Scandinavica* 138, no. 5 (2018): 368–378. https://doi
.org/10.1111/acps.12904.

Erritzoe, David, Balazs Sziget, Amanda Fielding, Robin
Carhart-Harris, and David Nutt. "Self-Blinding Microdose
Study." Accessed July 28, 2021. https://selfblinding
-microdose.org/sign-up.

Fadiman, James and Sophia Korb. "Drugs and Supplements."
MicrodosingPhyschedlics.com. https://sites.google.com/view
/microdosingpsychedelics/drugs-and-supplements.
Accessed October 8, 2021.

Fadiman, James and Sophia Korb. "Microdosing Psychedelics." In *Advances in Psychedelic Medicine: State-of-the-Art Therapeutic Applications,* edited by Michael J. Winkelman, 318–335. Santa Barbara: Praeger, 2019a.

Fadiman, James and Sophia Korb. "Microdosing: The Phenomenon, Research Results and Startling Surprises." *Psychedelic Science* 2017. April 21, 2017, Oakland. https://2017.psychedelicscience.org/conference/inter disciplinary/microdosing-the-phenomenon,-research -results,-and-startling-surprises.

Fadiman, James and Sophia Korb. "Might Microdosing Psychedelics Be Safe and Beneficial? An Initial Exploration." *Journal of Psychoactive Drugs* 51, no. 2 (2019b): 118–122. https://doi.org/10.1080/02791072.2019.1593561.

Fadiman, James. "Microdose Research: Without Approvals, Control Groups, Double Blinds, Staff, or Funding." *Microdose Research,* 2016. https://www.researchgate.net /publication/308138461_Microdose_research_without _approvals_control_groups_double_blinds_staff_or_funding.

Fadiman, James. Emails to Carlton J. Spotswood, March 2021.

Fadiman, James. Emails to Torsten Passie, July–Sept 2018.

Fadiman, James. *The Psychedelic Explorer's Guide: Safe, Therapeutic, and Sacred Journeys.* Rochester, VT: Park Street Press, 2011.

Family, Neiloufar, Emeline L. Maillet, Luke T. J. Williams, Erwin Krediet, Robin L. Carhart-Harris, Tim M. Williams, Charles D. Nichols, Daniel J. Goble, and Shlomi Raz. "Safety, Tolerability, Pharmacokinetics, and Pharmacodynamics of Low Dose Lysergic Acid Diethylamide (LSD) in Healthy

Older Volunteers." *Psychopharmacology (Berlin, Germany)* 237, no. 3 (2020): 841–853. https://doi.org/10.1007/s00213 -019-05417-7.

Fanciullacci, M., E. Del Bene, G. Franchi, and F. Sicuteri. "Brief Report: Phantom Limb Pain: Sub-Hallucinogenic Treatment with Lysergic Acid Diethylamide (LSD-25)." *Headache* 17, no. 3 (1977): 118–119. https://doi.org/10.1111/j.1526-4610.1977 .hed1703118.x.

Ferguson, James M. "SSRI Antidepressant Medications: Adverse Effects and Tolerability." *Primary Care Companion to the Journal of Clinical Psychiatry* 3, no. 1 (2001): 22–27. https://doi.org:10.4088/PCC.v03n0105.

Ferriss, Tim. "The Psychedelic Explorer's Guide: Microdosing, Mind Enhancing Methods, and More." *The Tim Ferriss Show*. Podcast. March 21, 2015. https://tim.blog/2015/03/21 /james-fadiman/.

Flanagan, Thomas W., and Charles D. Nichols. "Psychedelics as Anti-Inflammatory Agents." *International Review of Psychiatry* 30, no. 4 (2018): 363–375. https://doi.org/10.1080 /09540261.2018.1481827.

Flanagan, Thomas W., Melanie N. Sebastian, Diana M. Battalagia, Timothy P. Foster, Stephania A. Cormier, Charles D. Nichols. "5-HT2 Receptor Activation Alleviates Airway Inflammation and Structural Remodeling in a Chronic Mouse Asthma Model." *Life Sciences* 236 (2019): 116790– 116790. https://doi.org/10.1016/j.lfs.2019.116790.

Flanagan, Thomas W., Melanie N. Sebastian, Diana M. Battalagia, Timothy P. Foster, Stephania A. Cormier, Charles D. Nichols. "5-HT2 Receptor Activation Alleviates Airway Inflammation Activation of 5-HT2 Receptors

Reduces Inflammation in Vascular Tissue and Cholesterol Levels in High-Fat Diet-Fed Apolipoprotein E Knockout Mice. *Scientific Reports* 9, no. 1 (2019): 1–10. https://doi .org/10.1038/s41598-019-49987-0.

Fookes, Carmen. "Sumatriptan: 7 Things You Should Know." *Drugs.com.* Last updated July 5, 2021. https://www.drugs .com/tips/sumatriptan-patient-tips.

Forstmann, Matthia and Christina Sagioglo. "How Psychedelic Researchers' Self-Admitted Substance Use and Their Association with Psychedelic Culture Affect People's Perceptions of Their Scientific Integrity and the Quality of Their Research." *Public Understanding of Science (Bristol, England)* 30, no. 3 (2020): 302–318. https://doi .org/10.1177/0963662520981728.

Frederking, W. "The Use of Narcotics (Mescaline and Lysergic Acid Diethylamide) in Psychotherapy." *Psyche* 7, no. 6 (1953), 342.

Gilman, Ken. "Monoamine Oxidase Inhibitors: A Review Concerning Dietary Tyramine and Drug Interactions." *PsychoTropical Commentaries* 1, no. 1 (2017): 105.

Gliedman, Lester H., Earl H. Nash Jr., Stanley D. Imber, Anthony R. Stone, and Jerome D. Frank. "Reduction of Symptoms by Pharmacologically Inert Substances and by Short-Term Psychotherapy." *A.M.A. Archives of Neurology and Psychiatry* 79, no. 3 (1958): 345–351. https://doi .org/10.1001/archneurpsyc.1958.02340030109018.

Greiner, T., N. R. Burch, and R. Edelberg. "Psychopathology and Psychophysiology of Minimal LSD-25 Dosage; a Preliminary Dosage-Response Spectrum."*A.M.A. Archives of*

Neurology and Psychiatry 79, no. 2 (1958): 208–210. https://
doi.org/10.1001/archneurpsyc.1958.02340020088016.

Greiner, T., N. R. Burch, and R. Edelberg. "Threshold Doses of
LSD in Human Subjects." *Federation Proceedings* 16, no. 1
(1957): 303.

Griffiths, Ronald R., Michael A. Carducci, Annie Umbricht,
William A. Richards, Brian D. Richards, Mary P.
Cosimano, and Margaret A. Klinedinst. "Psilocybin
Produces Substantial and Sustained Decreases in
Depression and Anxiety in Patients with Life-Threatening
Cancer: A Randomized Double-Blind Trial." *Journal of
Psychopharmacology* 30, no. 12 (2016): 1181–1197. https://
doi.org/10.1177/0269881116675513.

Grinspoon, L., and J. B. Bakalar. *Psychedelic Drugs
Reconsidered.* New York: Basic Books, 1979.

Grof, S. *LSD Psychotherapy* (4th edition). Ben Lomond, CA:
MAPS Publishing, 1980.

Grumman, Christina, Kerstin Henkel, Simon D. Brandt,
Alexander Stratford, Torsten Passie, and Volker Auwärter.
"Pharmacokinetics and Subjective Effects of 1P-LSD in
Humans After Oral and Intravenous Administration." *Drug
Testing and Analysis* 12, no. 8 (2020): 1144–1153. https://doi
.org/10.1002/dta.2821.

Halberstadt, Adam L., and Mark A. Geyer. "Multiple Receptors
Contribute to the Behavioral Effects of Indoleamine
Hallucinogens." *Neuropharmacology* 61, no. 3 (2011): 364–
381. https://doi.org/10.1016/j.neuropharm.2011.01.017.

Harman, Willis W., Robert H. McKim, Robert E. Mogar, James
Fadiman, and Myron J. Stolaroff. "Psychedelic Agents in

Creative Problem-Solving: A Pilot Study." *Psychological Reports* 19, no, 1 (1966): 211–227. https://doi.org/10.2466 /pr0.1966.19.1.211.

Hartman, Shelby and Madison Margolin. "The Case for Macrodosing." *Rolling Stone*. December 12, 2020. https:// www.rollingstone.com/culture/culture-features /microdosing-macrodosing-psychedelics-psilocybin-lsd -trip-1100851.

Hartogsohn, Ido. "Set and Setting, Psychedelics and the Placebo Response: An Extra-Pharmacological Perspective on Psychopharmacology." *SAGE Publications* 30, np. 2 (2016): 1259–1267. https://doi .org/10.1177/0269881116677852.

Hartogsohn, Ido. *American Trip: Set, Setting, and the Psychedelic Experience in the Twentieth Century*. The MIT Press, 2020.

Hasler F., D. Bourquin, R. Brenneisen, T. Bar, and Franz X. Vollenweider. "Renal Excretion Profiles of Psilocin Following Oral Administration of Psilocybin: A Controlled Study in Man." *Journal of Pharmaceutical and Biomedical Analysis*. 30, no. 2 (2002): 331–9. https://doi.org/10.1016 /s0731-7085(02)00278-9.

Hasler Felix. "Untersuchungen Zur Human Pharmakokinetik von Psilocybin." Dissertation. University of Berne (Switzerland), Berne, 1997.

Hasler, Felix, Ullrike Grimberg, Marco A. Benz, Theo Huber, and Franz X. Vollenweider. "Acute Psychological and Physiological Effects of Psilocybin in Healthy Humans: A Double-Blind, Placebo-Controlled Dose-Effect Study." *Psychopharmacology* 172, no. 2 (2004): 145–156. https://doi .org/10.1007/s00213-003-1640-6.

Hasler, Felix., D. Bourquin, R. Brenneisen, T. Bar, and Franz X. Vollenweider. "Determination of Psilocin and 4-Hydroxyindole-3-Acetic Acid in Plasma by HPLC-ECD and Pharmacokinetic Profiles of Oral and Intravenous Psilocybin in Man." *Pharmaceutica Acta Helvetiae* 72, no. 3 (1997): 175–84. https://doi.org/10.1016/S0031 -6865(97)00014-9.

Helman, Cecil G. "Placebos and Nocebos: The Cultural Construction of Belief." In *Understanding the Placebo Effect in Complementary Medicine*, edited by David Peters. London: Churchill Livingstone, 2001.

Hendin, Holly M., and Andrew D. Penn. "An Episode of Mania Following Self-Reported Ingestion of Psilocybin Mushrooms in a Woman Previously Not Diagnosed with Bipolar Disorder: A Case Report." *Bipolar Disorders* (2021). https:// doi.org/10.1111/bdi.13095.

Hernández, Medardo, María Victoria Barahona, Ulf Simonsen, Paz Recio, Luis Rivera, Ana Cristina Martínez, Albino García-Sacristán, Luis M Orensanz, and Dolores Prieto. "Characterization of the 5-Hydroxytryptamine Receptors Mediating Contraction in the Pig Isolated Intravesical Ureter." *British Journal of Pharmacology* 138, no.1 (2003): 137–144. https://doi.org/10.1038/sj.bjp.0705019.

Hoffer, A., and H. Osmond. *Hallucinogens*. New York: Academic Press, 1967.

Hofmann, A. "LSD: Completely Personal." *Newsletter of the Multidisciplinary Association for Psychedelics Studies MAPS* 6, no. 3 (1996).

Hofmann, A. *LSD: My Problem Child*. San Jose: Multi-disciplinary Association for Psychedelic Studies, 2005.

Hofmann, A., A. Frey, H. Ott, T. Petr Zilka, and F. Troxler. "Elucidation of the Structure and the Synthesis of Psilocybin." *Experientia* 14, no. 11 (1958): 397. https://doi .org/10.1007/BF02160424.

Hofmann, A., R. Heim, A. Brack, and H. Kobel. "Psilocybin, a Psychotropic Substance from the Mexican Mushroom Psilicybe Mexicana Heim." *Experientia* 14, no. 3 (1958): 107. https://doi.org/10.1007/BF02159243.

Horder, Jamie, Paul Matthews, and Robert Waldmann. "Placebo, Prozac and PLoS: Significant Lessons for Psychopharmacology." *SAGE Publications* 25, no. 10 (2011). https://doi.org/10.1177/0269881110372544.

Horowitz, Michael. "Albert Hofmann." *High Times*. July 1, 1976. https://archive.hightimes.com/article/1976/7/1/albert -hofmann.

House, R. V., P. T. Thomas, and H. N. Bhargava. "Immunological Consequences of In Vitro Exposure to Lysergic Acid Diethylamide (LSD)." *Immunopharmacology and Immunotoxicology* 16, no. 1 (1994): 23. https://doi.org/10 .3109/08923979409029898.

Hutcheson, Joshua D., Vincent Setola, Bryan L. Roth, and W. David Merryman. "Serotonin Receptors and Heart Valve Disease–It Was Meant 2B." *Pharmacology and Therapeutics* 132, no. 2 (2011): 146–157. https://doi.org/10.1016/j .pharmthera.2011.03.008.

Hutten, Nadia R. P. W., Natasha L. Mason, Patrick C. Dolder, Eef L. Theunissen, Matthias E. Liechti, Amanda Feilding, Johannes G. Ramaekers, and Kim P. C. Kuypers. "Mood and Cognition After Administration of Low LSD Doses in Healthy Volunteers: A Placebo Controlled Dose-Effect

Finding Study." *European Neuropsychopharmacology* 41, (2020a): 81–91. https://doi.org/10.1016/j.euroneuro .2020.10.002.

Hutten, Nadia R., Natasha L. Mason, Patrick C. Dolder, and Kim P. C. Kuypers. "Motives and Side-Effects of Microdosing With Psychedelics Among Users." *The International Journal of Neuropsychopharmacology* 22, no. 7 (2019): 426–434. htpps://doi.org/10.1093/ijnp/pyz029.

Hutten, Nadia R. P. W., Natasha L. Mason, Patrick C. Dolder, Eef L. Theunissen, Matthias E. Liechti, Amanda Feilding, Johannes G. Ramaekers, and Kim P. C. Kuypers. "Cognitive and Subjective Effects of Different Low 'Micro' Doses of LSD in a Placebo-Controlled Study." *European Neuropsychopharmacology* 31 (2020b): S63–S64. https://doi .org/10.1016/j.euroneuro.2019.12.086.

Hutten, Nadia R. P. W., Natasha L. Mason, Patrick C. Dolder, Eef L. Theunissen, Friederike Holze, Matthias E. Liechti, Nimmy Varghese, Anne Eckert, Amanda Feilding, Johannes G. Ramaekers, and Kim P. C. Kuypers. "Low Doses of LSD Acutely Increase Bdnf Blood Plasma Levels in Healthy Volunteers." *American Chemical Society Pharmacological Translation Science* 4, no. 2 (2020c): 461–466. https://doi .org/10.1021/acsptsci.0c00099.

Hutten, Nadia R. P. W., Natasha L. Mason, Patrick C. Dolder, and Kim P. C. Kuypers. "Self-rated Effectiveness of Micro-dosing With Psychedelics for Mental and Physical Health Problems Among Microdosers." *Frontiers in Psychiatry* 13, no. 10 (2019): 672. https://doi.org/10.3389/fpsyt.2019 .00672.

Hysek C., Y. Schmid, A. Rickli, et al. "Carvedilol Inhibits the Cardiostimulant and Thermogenic Effects of MDMA in Humans." *Br J Pharmacol* 166 no. 8 (2012): 2277-2288. doi:10.1111/j.1476-5381.2012.01936.x.

Hysek, Cédric M et al. "Effects of the α_2-adrenergic Agonist Clonidine on the Pharmacodynamics and Pharmacokinetics of 3,4-methylenedioxymethamphetamine in Healthy Volunteers." *The Journal of Pharmacology and Experimental Therapeutics* 340, no. 2 (2012): 286-94. doi:10.1124/jpet.111.188425.

Idell, R. D., G. Florova, A. A. Komissarov, S. Shetty, R. B. S. Girard, and S. Idell. "The Fibrinolytic System: A New Target for Treatment of Depression with Psychedelics." *Medical Hypotheses* 100, (2017): 46–53. https://doi.org/10.1016/j.mehy.2017.01.013.

Isbell, Harris, A. B. Wolbach, and E. J. Miner. "Cross Tolerance Between LSD and Psilocybin." *Psychopharmacologia* 2 (1961): 147–159. https://doi.org/10.1007/BF00407974.

Isbell, Harris and D. R. Jasinski. "A Comparison of LSD-25 With (-)-Delta-9-trans-tetrahydrocannabinol (THC) and Attempted Cross Tolerance Between LSD and THC." *Psychopharmacologia* 14, no. 2 (1969): 115. https:/doi.org/10.1007/BF00403684.

Isbell, Harris, R. E. Belleville, H. F. Fraser, Abraham Wikler, and C. R. Logan. "Studies on Lysergic Acid Diethylamide (LSD-25). I. Effects in Former Morphine Addicts and Development of Tolerance During Chronic Intoxication." *A.M.A. Archives of Neurology and Psychiatry* 76, no. 5 (1956): 468–478. https://doi.org/10.1001/archneurpsyc.1956.023303290012002.

Isbell, Harris. "Comparison of the Reactions Induced by Psilocybin and LSD-25 in Man.". *Psychopharmacologia* 1, (1959): 29–38. https://doi.org/10.1007/BF00408109.

Janikian, Michelle. *Your Psilocybin Mushroom Companion: An Informative Easy-to-Use Guide to Understanding Magic Mushrooms.* Berkeley, CA: Ulysses Press, 2019.

Jerome, Lisa. "Psilocybin: Investigator's Brochure." *Multidisciplinary Association for Psychedelic Studies.* 2007. https://maps.org/research-archive/psilo/psilo_ib.pdf.

Johansen, Pal-Ørjan and Teri Suzanne Krebs. "Psychedelics Not Linked to Mental Health Problems or Suicidal Behavior: A Population Study." *Journal of Psychopharmacology (Oxford, England)* 29, no. 3 (2015): 270–279. https://doi.org/10.1177/0269881114568039.

Johnson, Matthew W., and Roland R. Griffiths. "Potential Therapeutic Effects of Psilocybin." *Neurotherapeutics* 14, no. 3 (2017): 734–740. https://doi.org/10.1007/s13311-017-0542-y.

Johnson, Matthew W., R. Andrew Sewell, and Ronald R. Griffiths. "Psilocybin Dose-Dependently Causes Delayed, Transient Headaches in Healthy Volunteers." *Drug and Alcohol Dependence* 123, no. 1 (2012): 132–140. https://doi.org/10.1016/j.drugalcdep.2011.10.029.

Johnson, Matthew W., Roland R. Griffiths, Peter S. Hendricks, and Jack E. Henningfield. "The Abuse Potential of Medical Psilocybin According to the 8 Factors of the Controlled Substances Act." *Neuropharmacology* 142 (2018): 143–166. https://doi.org/10.1016/j.neuropharm.2018.05.012.

Johnson, Matthew W., William A. Richards, and Roland R. Griffiths. "Human Hallucinogen Research: Guidelines for Safety." *Journal of Psychopharmacology (Oxford)* 22, no. 6 (2008): 603–620. https://doi.org/10.1177/0269881108093587.

Johnstad, Petter Grahl. "Powerful Substances in Tiny Amounts: An Interview Study of Psychedelic Microdosing." *Nordic Studies on Alcohol and Drugs* 35, no. 1 (2018): 39–51. https://doi.org/10.1177/1455072517753339.

Jones, Simone Vann, and Ilias Kounatidis. "Nuclear Factor-Kappa B and Alzheimer Disease, Unifying Genetic and Environmental Risk Factors From Cell to Humans." *Frontiers in Immunology* 11 (2017): 1805. https://doi.org/10.3389/fimmu.2017.01805.

Kaertner, L. S., M. B. Steinborn, H. Kettner, M. J. Spriggs, L. Roseman, T. Buchborn, M. Balaet, C. Timmermann, D. Erritzoe, and R. L. Carhart-Harris. "Positive Expectations Predict Improved Mental-Health Outcomes Linked to Psychedelic Microdosing." *Scientific Reports* 11, no. 1 (2021): 1941. https://doi.org/10.1038/s41598-021-81446-7.

Kaplan, Harold I., Benjamin J. Sadock, and Jack A. Grebb. *Kaplan and Sadock's Synopsis of Psychiatry: Behavioral Sciences, Clinical Psychiatry 7th Edition.* Philadelphia: Williams and Wilkins Co., 1994.

Kaptchuk, T. J. "Powerful Placebo: The Dark Side of the Randomised Controlled Trial." *The Lancet (British Edition)* 351, no. 9117 (1998): 1722–1725. https://doi.org/10.1016/S0140-6736(97)10111-8.

Karst, Matthias, John H. Halpern, Michael Bernateck, and Torsten Passie. "The Non-hallucinogen 2-Bromo-Lysergic Acid Diethylamide As Preventative Treatment for Cluster

Headache: An Open, Non-randomized Case Series." *Cephalalgia* 30, no. 9 (2010): 1140–1144. https://doi .org/10.1177/0333102410363490.

Kast, E. "Attenuation of Anticipation: A Therapeutic Use of Lysergic Acid Diethylamide." *Psychiatric Quarterly* 41, no. 4 (1967), 646.

Kast, E. "LSD and the Dying Patient." *The Chicago Medical School Quarterly,* 26, no. 2 (1966): 80.

Kast, E. C., and V. J. Collins. "Study of Lysergic Acid Diethylamide as an Analgesic Agent." *Anesthesia and Analgesia* 43 (1964): 285.

Keeler, Martin H. "Chlorpromazine Antagonism of Psilocybin Effect." *International Journal of Neuropsychiatry* 3, (1967): 66–71.

Kirsch Irving. "Challenging Received Wisdom: Antidepressants and the Placebo Effect." *McGill Journal of Medicine 11*, no. 2 (2008), 219–222.

Kirsch, Irving, and G. Sapirstein. "Listening to Prozac but Hearing Placebo: A Meta-analysis of Antidepressant Medication." *Prevention and Treatment* 1, no. 2 (1998). https://doi.org/10.1037/1522-3736.1.1.12a.

Kirsch, Irving, Brett J. Deacon, Tania B. Huedo-Medina, Alan Scoboria, Thomas J. Moore, and Blair T. Johnson. "Initial Severity and Antidepressant Benefits: A Meta-analysis of Data Submitted to the Food and Drug Administration." *PLoS Medicine* 5, no. 2 (2008): e45. https://doi.org/10.1371/journal .pmed.0050045.

Kirsch, Irving. "Antidepressants and the Placebo Effect." *Zeitschrift für Psychologie* 222, no. 3 (2015): 128–134. https://doi.org/10.1027/2151-2604/a000176.

Knight, Anthony R., Anil Misra, Kathleen QUirk, Karen Benwell, Dean Revell, Guy Kennett, and Mike Bikcerdike. "Pharmacological Characterisation of the Agonist Radioligand Binding Site of 5-HT 2A, 5-HT 2B and 5-HT 2C Receptors." *Naunyn-Schmiedeberg's Archives of Pharmacology* 370, no. 2 (2004): 114–123. https://doi.org/10.1007/s00210-004-0951-4.

Koch, Bryce. Personal Communication. May 29, 2021.

Köhler-Forsberg, O., C. N. Lydholm, C. Hjorthøj, M. Nordentoft, O. Mors, and M. E. Benros. "Efficacy of Anti-inflammatory Treatment on Major Depressive Disorder or Depressive Symptoms: Meta-analysis of Clinical Trials." *Acta Psychiatrica Scandinavica* 139, no. 5 (2019): 404–419. https://doi.org/10.1111/acps.13016.

Koslow, Tyler. "SSRI and LSD Interactions, Plus Shrooms and More: Why Taking Psychedelics While on Antidepressants Could Make Treatment Ineffective." *Double Blind.* Last updated June 2, 2020. https://doubleblindmag.com/how-psychedelics-contraindicate-with-ssris.

Krebs, Teri S., and Pål-Ørjan Johansen. "Psychedelics and Mental Health: A Population Study." *PloS One*, 8, no. 8 (2013): e63972. https://doi.org/10.1371/journal.pone.0063972.

Krippner, Stanley. "Psychedelic Drugs and Creativity." *Journal of Psychoactive Drugs* 17, no. 4 (1985): 235–246. https://doi.org/10.1080/02791072.1985.10524328.

Kroenke, K., R. L. Spitzer, and J. B. W. Williams. "The PHQ-9—Validity of a Brief Depression Severity Measure." *Journal of General Internal Medicine* 16 (2001): 606–13.

Kuromaru, S., S. Okada, M. Hanada, Y. Kasahara, and K. Sakamoto. "The Effect of LSD on the Phantom Limb Phenomenon." *The Journal-Lancet* 87, no. 1 (1967): 22.

Kuypers, Kim P. C. "The Therapeutic Potential of Microdosing Psychedelics in Depression." *Therapeutic Advances in Psychopharmacology* 10 (2020): 1–15. https://doi .org/10.1177/2045125320950567.

Kuypers, Kim P. C., Livia Ng, David Erritzoe, Gitte M. Knudsen, Charles D. Nichols, David E. Nichols, Luca Pani, Anaïs Soula, and David Nutt. "Microdosing Psychedelics: More Questions Than Answers? An Overview and Suggestions for Future Research." *Journal of Psychopharmacology (Oxford)* 33, no. 9 (2019): 1039–1057. https://doi.org/10.1177/02698811198 57204.

Lake, C. R., A. L. Stirba, R. E. Kinneman Jr., B. Carlson, and H. C. Holloway. "Mania Associated with LSD Ingestion." *The American Journal of Psychiatry* 138, no. 11 (1981): 1508–1509. https://doi.org/10.1176/ajp.138.11.1508.

Lea, Toby, Nicole Amada, and Henrik Jungaberle. "Psychedelic Microdosing: A Subreddit Analysis." *Journal of Psychoactive Drugs,* 52, no. 2 (2020a): 1–12. https://doi.org/10.1080/02791 072.2019.1683260.

Lea, Toby, Nicole Amada, Henrik Jungaberle, Henrike Schecke, and Michael Klein. "Microdosing Psychedelics: Motivations, Subjective Effects and Harm Reduction." *The International Journal of Drug Policy* 75 (2020b): 102600. https://doi.org/10 .1016/j.drugpo.2019.11.008.

Lea, Toby, Nicole Amada, Henrik Jungaberle, Henrike Schecke, Norbert Scherbaum, and Michael Klein. "Perceived Outcomes of Psychedelic Microdosing As Self-managed Therapies for Mental and Substance Use Disorders." *Psychopharmacology (Berlin, Germany)* 237, no. 5 (2020c): 1521–1532. https://doi.org/10.1007/s00213-020-05477-0.

Leuchter, Andrew F., Aimee M. Hunter, Molly Tartter, and Ian A. Cook. " Role of Pill-Taking, Expectation and Therapeutic Alliance in the Placebo Response in Clinical Trials for Major Depression." *British Journal of Psychiatry* 205, no. 6 (2018): 443–449. https://doi.org/10.1192/bjp.bp.113.140343.

Lugo-Radillo, Augustin, and Jorge Luis Cortes-Lopez. "Long-Term Amelioration of OCD Symptoms in a Patient with Chronic Consumption of Psilocybin-Containing Mushrooms." *Journal of Psychoactive Drugs* 53, no. 2 (2021): 1–3. https://doi.org/10.1080/02791072.2020.1849879.

Ly, Calvin, Alexandr C. Greb, Lindsay P. Cameron, Jonathan M. Wong, Eden V. Barragan, Paige C. Wilson, Kyle F. Burbach, et al. "Psychedelics Promote Structural and Functional Neural Plasticity." *Cell Reports (Cambridge)* 23, no. 11 (2018: 3170–3182. https://doi.org/10.1016/j.cel rep.2018.05.022.

MacLean, Katherine A., Matthew W. Johnson, and Ronald R. Griffiths. "Mystical Experiences Occasioned by the Hallucinogen Psilocybin Lead to Increases in the Personality Domain of Openness." *Journal of Psychopharmacology (Oxford)* 25, no. 11 (2011): 1453–1461. https://doi.org/10.1177/0269881111420188.

Madsen, Martin K., Patrick M. Fisher, Daniel Burmester, Agnete Dyssengaard, Dea S. Stenbaek, Sara Kristiansen, Sys

S. Johansen, et al. "Psychedelic Effects of Psilocybin Correlate With Serotonin 2A Receptor Occupancy and Plasma Psilocin Levels." *Neuropsychopharmacology* 44, no. 7 (2019): 1328–1334. https://doi.org/10.1038/s41386-019-0324-9.

Malcolm, Benjamin J., and Kimberly Tallian. "Essential Oil of Lavender in Anxiety Disorders: Ready for Prime Time?" *The Mental Health Clinician*, vol. 7, no. 4, 2017, pp. 147–155.

Malcolm, Benjamin. "Antidepressant and Psychedelic Combinations: A Guide to Risks & Discontinuation Times." *Spirit Pharmacist*. November 2019. https://psychedelic network.org.uk/antidepressant-and-psychedelic -combinations-a-guide-to-risks-discontinuation-times.

Malcolm, Benjamin. "Antidepressant and Psychedelic Drug Interaction Chart." *Psychedelic School*. August 2020. https://s3.amazonaws.com/kajabi-storefronts-production /sites/111358/downloads/NU3bVJNgTJeI6G8M8YH4 _Antidepressant_PsychedelicsChart_PsychedelicSchool.pdf.

Malcolm, Benjamin and Kelan Thomas. "Serotonin Toxicity of Serotonergic Psychedelics." *Psychopharmacology* (2021). https://doi.org/10.1007/s00213-021-05876-x.

Maslej, Marta M., Toshiaki A. Furukawa, Andrea Cipriani, Paul W. Andrews, Marcos Sanches, Anneka Tomlinson, and Constantin Volkmann, et al. "Individual Differences in Response to Antidepressants: A Meta-analysis of Placebo-Controlled Randomized Clinical Trials." *JAMA Psychiatry* 78, no. 5 (2021): 490–497. https://doi.org/10.1001/jama psychiatry.2020.4564.

Mason, N. L., K. P. C. Kuyers, F. Muller, D. H. Y. Tse, S. W. Toenees, N. R. P. W. Hutten, J. F. A. Jansen, et al. "Me, Myself, Bye: Regional Alterations in Glutamate and the Experience of Ego

Dissolution with Psilocybin." *Neuropsychopharmacology* 45, (2020): 2003–2011. https://doi.org/10.1038/s4386-020-0718-8.

Matsumoto, J., and M. Jouvet. "Effects of Reserpine, Dopa and 5-Htp on the 2 Sleep States." *Comptes Rendus Des Séances De La Société De Biologie Et De Ses Filiales* 158, (1964): 2137–2140.

Matsushima Yoshihiro, Osamu Shirota, Ruri Kikura-Hanajiri, Yukihiro Goda, and Fumio Eguchi. "Effects of *Psilocybe argentipes* on Marble-Burying Behavior in Mice." *Bioscience, Biotechnology, and Biochemistry* 73, no. 8 (2009): 1866–1868. https://doi.org/10.1271/bbb.90095.

McCorvy, John D., Daniel Wacker, Sheng Wang, Bemnat Agegnehu, Jing Liu, Katherine Lansu, Alexandra R. Tribo, et al. "Structural Determinants of 5-HT2B Receptor Activation and Biased Agonism." *Nature Structural and Molecular Biology* 25, no. 9 (2018): 787–796. https://doi.org/10.1038/s41594-018-0116-7.

Melander, Hans, Jane Ahlqvist-Rastad, Gertie Meijer, and Bjorn Beerman. "Evidence B(i)ased Medicine—Selective Reporting From Studies Sponsored by the Pharmaceutical Industry: Review of Studies in New Drug Applications." *British Medical Journal* 326, no. 7400 (2003): 1171–1173. https://doi.org/10.1136/bmj.326.7400.1171.

Microdosingpsychedelics. "Drugs and Supplements." *Microdosingpsychedelics.com.* Accessed July 29, 2021. https://sites.google.com/view/microdosingpsychedelics/drugs-and-supplements.

Miller, Andrew H. Miller, Vladimir Maletic, and Charles L. Raison. "Inflammation and Its Discontents: The Role of Cytokines in the Pathophysiology of Major Depression."

Biological Psychiatry 65, no. 9 (2009): 732–741. https://doi
.org/10.1016/j.biopsych.2008.11.029.

Miyazaki, Katsuhiko, Kayoko W. Miyazaki, and Kenji Doya.
"The Role of Serotonin in the Regulation of Patience and
Impulsivity." *Molecular Neurobiology* 45, no. 2 (2012):
213–224. https://doi.org/10.1007/s12035-012-8232-6.

Moerman, Daniel E. *Meaning, Medicine and the "Placebo Effect."*
Cambridge: Cambridge University Press, 2002.

Moerman, Daniel E., and Wayne B. Jones. "Deconstructing the
Placebo Effect and Finding the Meaning Response." *Annals
of Internal Medicine* 136, no. 6 (2002): 471. https://doi
.org/10.7326/0003-4819-136-6-200203190-00011.

Moreno, F. A., C. B. Wiegand, E. K. Taitano, and P. L. Delgado.
"Safety, Tolerability, and Efficacy of Psilocybin in 9 Patients
With Obsessive-Compulsive Disorder." *The Journal of
Clinical Psychiatry* 67, no. 11 (2006): 1735–1740. https://doi
.org/10.4088/jcp.v67n1110.

Moreno, F. A., P. L. Delgado. "Hallucinogen-Induced Relief
of Obsessions and Compulsions." *The American Journal of
Psychiatry* 154, no. 7 (1997): 1037–1038. https://doi
.org/10.1176/ajp.154.7.1037b.

Morris, Hamilton. "Blood Spore." *Harper's Magazine.* Accessed
July 29, 2021. https://harpers.org/archive/2013/07/blood
-spore.

Morski, Lynn Marie. "Microdose Q&A with James Fadiman."
Plant Medicine Podcast. August 19, 2020. https://www
.plantmedicine.org/podcast/microdosing-james-fadiman.

Murphy, Robin J., Rachel L. Sumner, William Evans, David
Menkes, Ingo Lambrecht, Rhys Ponton, Frederick Sundram,

et al. "MDLSD: Study Protocol for a Randomised, Double-Masked, Placebo-Controlled Trial of Repeated Microdoses of LSD in Healthy Volunteers." *Trials* 22, no. 1 (2021): 302. https://doi.org/10.1186/s13063-021-05243-3.

Muzio, J. N., H. P. Roffwarg, E. Kauffman. "Alterations in the Nocturnal Sleep Cycle Resulting From LSD." *Electroencephalography and Clinical Neurophysiology* 21, no. 4 (1966): 313–324. https://doi.org/10.1016/0013-4694(66)90037-x.

Nasrallah, Henry A. "Treatment Resistance Is a Myth!" *Current Psychiatry* 20, no. 3 (2021): 14–16, 28. https://doi.org/10.12788/cp.0105.

National Library of Medicine. "Lysergic Acid Diethylamide (LSD) as Treatment for Cluster Headache." *ClinicalTrials.gov*. Last updated April 20, 2021. https://clinicaltrials.gov/ct2/show/NCT03781128?term=LSD+for+Cluster+Headaches&draw=2&rank=1.

National Library of Medicine. "The Safety and Efficacy of Psilocybin in Participants With Type 2 Bipolar Disorder (BP-II) Depression."*ClinicalTrials.gov*. Last updated March 3, 2021. https://clinicaltrials.gov/ct2/show/NCT04433845?term=psilocybin&cond=Bipolar+Depression&draw=2&rank=1.

Nau, Felix Jr., Bangning Yu, David Martin, and Charles D. Nichols. "Serotonin 5-HT2A Receptor Activation Blocks TNF-α Mediated Inflammation In Vivo." *Public Library of Science One* 2, no. 8 (2013): e75426. https://doi.org/10.1371/journal.pone.0075426.

Nau, Felix Jr., Justin Miller, Jordy Saravia, Terry Ahlert, Banging Yu, Kyle I. Happel, Stephania A. Cormier, and Charles D. Nichols. "Serotonin 5-HT2 Receptor Activation

Prevents Allergic Asthma in a Mouse Model." *American Journal of Physiology-Lung Cellular and Molecular Physiology* 308, no. 2 (2015): L191–L198. https://doi.org/10.1152/ajplung.0038.2013.

Nayak, Sandeep, Natalie Gukasyan, Frederick Streeter Barrett, Earth Erowid, Fire Erowid, and Ronald R. Griffiths. "Classic Psychedelic Coadministration With Lithium, but Not Lamotrigine, Is Associated With Seizures: An Analysis of Online Psychedelic Experience Reports." *PsyArXiv*, 2021. https://doi.10.31234/odf.io7r726d.

Naylor, E. V., D. O. Antonuccio, M. Litt, G. E. Johnson, D. R. Spogen, R. Williams, C. McCarthy, M. M. Lu, D. C. Fiore et al. "Bibliotherapy as a Treatment for Depression in Primary Care." *Journal of Clinical Psychology in Medical Settings* 17, no. 3 (August 2010): 258–271. https://doi.org/10.1007/s10880-010-9207-2.

Nebigil, Canan G., Fabrice Jaffré, Nadia Messaddeq, Pierre Hickel, Laurent Monassier, Jean-Marie Launay, and Luc Maroteaux. "Overexpression of the Serotonin 5-HT2B Receptor in Heart Leads to Abnormal Mitochondrial Function and Cardiac Hypertrophy." *Circulation* 107 (2020): 3223–3229. https://doi.org/10.1161/01.CIR.0000074224.57016.01.

Nichols David E. "Psychedelics." *Pharmacological Reviews* 68, no. 2 (2016): 264–355. https://doi.org/10.1124/pr.115.011478.

Nutt, David [@ProfDavidNutt]. "DAVE Nicholls and I modelled this a few years ago and found it unlikely that even repeated microdosding would influence the 2b receptor enough. @Drug_Science" Twitter, 22 November 2020,

twitter.com/ProfDavidNutt/status/1330483039009
464320?s=20.

Ona, Genis, and Jose Carlos Bouso. "Potential Safety, Benefits,
and Influence of the Placebo Effect in Microdosing
Psychedelic Drugs: A Systematic Review." *Neuroscience and
Biobehavioral Reviews* 119 (2020): 194–203. https://doi
.org/10.1016/j.neubiorev.2020.09.035.

Orlova, Yulia, Paul Rizzoli, and Elizabeth Loder. "Association
of Coprescription of Triptan Antimigraine Drugs and
Selective Serotonin Reuptake Inhibitor or Selective
Norepinephrine Reuptake Inhibitor Antidepressants with
Serotonin Syndrome." *JAMA Neurology* 75, no. 5 (2018): 566.
https://doi.org/10.1001/jamaneurol.2017.5144.

Oss, O. T., and O. N. Oeric. *Psilocybin: Magic Mushroom
Grower's Guide: A Handbook for Psilocybin Enthusiasts*, 13–
77. Oakland: Quick American Publishing Company, 1993.

Pahnke, Walter Norman. "Drugs and Mysticism: An Analysis
of the Relationship Between Psychedelic Drugs and
Mystical Consciousness." Harvard University, Cambridge,
1963. http://www.maps.org/images/pdf/books/pahnke
/walter_pahnke_drugs_and_mysticism.pdf.

Panik, Kristine, and David E. Presti. "LSD." In *Handbook of
Medical Hallucinogens*, edited by Charles S. Grob and Jim
Grisby, 347–362. New York: Guilford Press, 2021.

Park, Lee C., and Lino Covi. "Nonblind Placebo Trial: An
Exploration of Neurotic Patients' Responses to Placebo
When Its Inert Content Is Disclosed." *Archives of General
Psychiatry* 12, no. 4 (1965): 36–45. https://doi.org/10.1001
/archpsyc.1965.01720340008002.

Passie, Torsten, John H. Halpern, Dirk O. Stichtenoth, Hinderk M. Emrich, and Annelie Hintzen. "The Pharmacology of Lysergic Acid Diethylamide: A Review." *CNS Neuroscience and Therapeutics* 14, no. 4 (2008): 295–314. https://doi.org/10.1111/j.1755-5949.2008.00059.x.

Passie, Torsten, Juergen Seifert, Udo Schneider, and Hinderk M. Emrich. "The Pharmacology of Psilocybin." *Addiction Biology* 7, no. 4 (2006): 357–364. https://doi.org/10.1080/135 5621021000005937.

Passie, Torsten. *The Science of Microdosing Psychedelics.* London: Psychedelic Press, 2019.

Penn, Andrew D., Janis Phelps, William E. Rosa, and Jean Watson. "Psychedelic-Assisted Psychotherapy Practices and Human Caring Science: Toward a Care-Informed Model of Treatment." *Journal of Humanistic Psychology* (2021). https://doi.org/10.1177/00221678211011013.

Petranker, Rotem, Thomas Anderson, and Norman Farb. "Psychedelic Research and the Need for Transparency: Polishing Alice's Looking Glass." *Frontiers in Psychology* 11 (2020): 1681. https://doi.org/10.3389/fpsyg.2020.01681.

Petranker, Rotem, Thomas Anderson, Larissa J. Maier, Monica J. Barratt, and Jason A. Ferris. "Microdosing Psychedelics: Subjective Benefits and Challenges, Substance Testing Behavior, and the Relevance of Intention." *Journal of Psychopharmacology,* (2020): 1–12. https://doi.org/10.1177/0269881120953994.

Pokorny, Thomas, Katrin H. Preller, Rainer Kraehenmann, Franz X. Vollenweider. "Modulatory Effect of the 5-HT1A Agonist Buspirone and the Mixed Non-hallucinogenic 5-HT1A/2A Agonist Ergotamine on

Psilocybin-Induced Psychedelic Experience." *European Neuropsychopharmacology* 26, no. 4 (2016): 756–766. https://doi.org/10.1016/j.euroneuro.2016.01.005.

Polito, Vincent, and Richard J. Stevenson. "A Systematic Study of Microdosing Psychedelics." *Public Library of Science One* 14, no. 2 (2019): e0211023. https://doi.org/10.1371/journal.pone.0211023.

Pollan, Michael. *How to Change Your Mind: What the New Science of Psychedelics Teaches Us About Consciousness, Dying, Addiction, Depression, and Transcendence.* New York: Penguin Press, 2018.

Pollock, Steven Hayden. "The Psilocybin Mushroom Pandemic." *Journal of Psychedelic Drugs* 7, no. 1 (1975): 73–84. https://doi.org/10.1080/02791072.1975.10472640.

Prochazkova, Luisa, Dominique P. Lippelt, Lorenza S. Colzato, Martin Kuchar, Zsuzsika Sjoerds, and Bernhard Hommel. "Exploring the Effect of Microdosing Psychedelics on Creativity in an Open-label Natural Setting." *Psychopharmacology (Berlin, Germany)* 235, no. 12 (2018): 3401–3413. https://doi.org/10.1007/s00213-018-5049-7.

Rabkin, J. G., J. S. Markowitz, J. Stewart, P. McGrath, W. Harrison, F. M. Quitkin, and D. F. Klein. "How Blind Is Blind? Assessment of Patient and Doctor Medication Guesses in a Placebo-Controlled Trial of Imipramine and Phenelzine." *Psychiatry Research* 19, no. 1 (1986): 75–56. https://doi.org/10.1016/0165-1781(86)90094-6.

Ramachandran, Vilayanaur, Chaipat Chunhara, Zeve Marcus, Timothy Furnish, and Albert Lin. "Relief From Intractable Phantom Pain by Combining Psilocybin and Mirror

Visual-Feedback (MVF)." *Neurocase* 24, no. 2 (2018): 105–110. https://doi.org/10.1080/13554794.2018.1468469.

Ramaekers, Johannes G., Nadia Hutten, Natasha L. Mason, Patrick Dolder, Eef L. Theunissen, Friederike Holze, Matthias E. Liechti, et al. "A Low Dose of Lysergic Acid Diethylamide Decreases Pain Perception in Healthy Volunteers." *Journal of Psychopharmacology (Oxford)* 35, no. 4 (2020): 398–405. https://doi.org/10.1177/0269881120 940937.

Raval, Nakuil, Annette Johansen, Lene Lundgaard Donovan, Nidia Fernandez Ros, Brice Ozenne, Hanne Demant Hansen, and Gitte Moos Knudsen. "A Single Dose of Psilocybin Increases Synaptic Density and Decreases 5-HT2A Receptor Density in the Pig Brain." *International Journal of Molecular Sciences* 22, no. 2 (2021): 835. https://doi.org/10.3390/ijms22020835.

Ross. S., and L. W. Buckalew. "Placebo Agentry: Assessment of Drug and Placebo Effects." In *Placebo: Theory, Research, and Mechanisms*, edited by Leonard White, Bernard Tursky, and Gary E. Schwartz. New York: The Guilford Press, 1985.

Rothman, Richard B., Michael H. Baumann, Jason E. Savage, Laura Rauser, Ace McBride, Sandra J. Hufeisen, and Bryan L. Roth. "Evidence for Possible Involvement of 5-HT(2B) Receptors in the Cardiac Valvulopathy Associated With Fenfluramine and Other Serotonergic Medications." *Circulation* 102, no. 23 (2000): 2836–2841. https://doi.org/10.1161/01.cir.102.23.2836.

Ruck, C. A., J. Bigwood, D. Staples, J. Ott, and R. G. Wasson. "Entheogens." *Journal of Psychedelic Drugs* 11, no. 1 (1979): 145.

Sadock, Benjamin J., and Virgina A. Sadock. *Synopsis of Psychiatry Tenth Edition*. Philadelphia: Lippincott Williams and Wilkins, 2007.

Sapirstein, Guy. "The Effectiveness of Placebos in the Treatment of Depression: A Meta-analysis." University of Connecticut, January 1995. https://opencommons.uconn .edu/dissertations/AAI9605497.

Schindler, Emmanuelle A. D., Christopher H. Gottschalk, Marsha J. Weil, Robert E. Shapiro, Douglas A. Wright, and Richard Andrew Sewell. "Indoleamine Hallucinogens in Cluster Headache: Results of the Clusterbusters Medication Use Survey. *Journal of Psychoactive Drugs* 47, no. 5 (2015): 372–381. https://doi.org/10.1080/02791072.2015.1107664.

Schindler, Emmanuelle A. D., R. Andrew Sewell, Christopher H. Gottschalk, Christina Luddy, L. Taylor Flynn, Hayley Lindsey, Brian P. Pittman, Nicholas V. Cozzi, and Deepak C. D'Souza. "Exploratory Controlled Study of the Migraine-Suppressing Effects of Psilocybin." *Neurotherapeutics* 18, no. 1 (2021): 534–543. https://doi.org/10.1007/s13311-020 -00962-y.

Schott, Bjorn H., Constanze I. Seidenbecher, Sylvia Richter, Torsten Wüstenberg, Grazyna Debska-Vielhaber, Heike Schubert, Hans-Jochen Heinze, et al. "Genetic Variation of the Serotonin 2a Receptor Affects Hippocampal Novelty Processing in Humans." *PloS One* 6, no. 1 (2011): e15984. https://doi.org/10.1371/journal.pone.0015984.

Schotte, Chris K. W., Bart Van Den Bossche, Dirk De Doncker, Stephan Claes, and Paul Cosyns. "A Biopsychosocial Model as a Guide for Psychoeducation and Treatment of

Depression." *Depression and Anxiety* 23, no. 5 (2006): 312–324. https://doi.org/10.1002/da.20177.

Setti, S. E., H. C. Hunsberger, and M. N. Reed. "Alterations in Hippocampal Activity and Alzheimer's Disease." *Translational Issues in Psychological Science* 3, no. 4 (2017): 348–356. https://doi.org/10.1037/tps0000124.

Sewell, R. Andrew, John H. Halpern, and Harrison G. Pope Jr. "Response of Cluster Headache to Psilocybin and LSD." *Neurology* 66, no. 12 (2006): 1920. https://doi.org/10.1212/01.wnl.0000219761.05466.43.

Shapiro, A. K., and L. A. Morris. "The Placebo Effect in Medical and Psychological Therapies." In *Handbook of Psychotherapy and Behavioral Change Second Edition*, edited by Sol L. Garfield. New York: Wiley, 1978.

Sicuteri, F. "Headache As Metonymy of Non Organic Central Pain." In *Headache: New Vistas*, 19–67. Florence: Biomedical Press, 1977.

Sicuteri, F. "Prophylactic Treatment of Migraine by Means of Lysergic Acid Derivatives." *Triangle* 67 (1963): 116–125.

Sigafoos, Jeff, Vanessa A. Green, Chaturi Edrisinha, and Giulio E. Lancioni. "Flashback to the 1960s: LSD in the Treatment of Autism." *Developmental Neurorehabilitation* 10, no. 1 (2006): 75–81. https://doi.org/10.1080/13638490601106277.

Simonsson, Otto, James D. Sexton, and Peter S. Hendricks. "Associations Between Lifetime Classic Psychedelic Use and Markers of Physical Health." *Journal of Psychopharmacology* 35, no. 4 (2021): 447–452. https://doi.org/10.1177/026988 1121996863.

Simpson, Carra A., Camerla Diaz-Arteche, Djamila Eliby, Orli S. Schwartz, Julian G. Simmons, and Caitlin S. M. Cowan. "The Gut Microbiota in Anxiety and Depression–A Systematic Review." *Clinical Psychology Review* 83 (2021): 101943. https://doi.org/10.1016/j.cpr.2020.101943.

Sinyor, Mark, Ayal Schaffer, and Anthony Levitt. "The Sequenced Treatment Alternatives to Relieve Depression (STARD) Trial: A Review." *Canadian Journal of Psychiatry* 55, no. 3 (2010): 126. https://doi.org/10.1177/07067437100 5500303.

Spitzer R. L., K. Kroenke, J. B. Williams, B. A. Löwe. "A Brief Measure for Assessing Generalized Anxiety Disorder: The GAD-7." *Archives of Internal Medicine* 166, no. 10 (May 2006): 1092–1097.

Stamets, Paul. "Psilocybin Mushrooms and the Mycology of Consciousness." *Psychedelic Science 2017.* April 23, 2017. https://2017.psychedelicscience.org/conference/inter disciplinary/psilocybin-mushrooms-and-the-mycology -of-consciousness.

Strassman, Rick. "Adverse Reactions to Psychedelic Drugs. A Review of the Literature." *The Journal of Nervous and Mental Disease* 172, no. 10 (1984): 577–95. https://doi.org/10 .1097/00005053-198410000-00001.

Studerus, Erich, Alex Gamma, Michael Kometer, and Franz X. Vollenrweider, "Prediction of Psilocybin Response in Healthy Volunteers." *PloS One* 7, no. 2 (2012): e30800. https://doi.org/10.1371/journal.pone.0030800.

Studerus, Erich, Michael Kometer, Felix Hasler, and Franz X. Vollenweider. "Acute, Subacute and Long-term Subjective Effects of Psilocybin in Healthy Humans: A Pooled Analysis of Experimental Studies." *Journal of Psychopharmacology (Oxford)* 25, no. 11 (2010): 1434–1452. https://doi.org/10.1177/0269881110382466.

Sullivan, Laura C., William P. Clarke, and Kelly A. Ber. "Atypical Antipsychotics and Inverse Agonism at 5-HT2 Receptors." *Current Pharmaceutical Design* 21, no. 26 (2015): 3732. https://doi.org/10.2174/1381612821666150605111236.

Suzuki, Keiko. "Three Cases of Acute Serotonin Syndrome due to Psilocybin Mushroom Poisoning." *Chudoku Kenkyu: Chudoku Kenkyukai Jun Kikanshi = the Japanese Journal of Toxicology* 29, no. 1 (2016): 33.

Szabo, Attila. "Effects of Psychedelics on Inflammation and Immunity." In *Advances in Psychedelic Medicine: State-of-the-Art Therapeutic Applications*, edited by Michael J. Winkelman and Ben Sessa, 193–213. Westport, CT: Praeger, 2019.

Szigeti, Balazs, Laura Kartner, Allan Blemings, Fernando Rosas, Amanda Feilding, David J. Nutt, Robin L. Carhart-Harris, and David Erritzoe. "Self-blinding Citizen Science to Explore Psychedelic Microdosing." *Elife* 2021, no. 10 (2021). https://doi.org/10.7554/eLife.62878.

TEDx Talks. "The Power of Addiction and the Addiction of Power: Gabor Maté at TEDxRio+20." *YouTube.* October 9, 2012. https://www.youtube.com/watch?v=66cYcSak6nE.

Thomas, Kelan, and Benjamin Malcolm. "Adverse Effects." In *Handbook of Medical Hallucinogens*, edited by Charles S. Grob and Jim Grisby, 347–362. New York: Guilford Press, 2021.

Thomas, Kelan. "Why Chronic Microdosing May Break Your Heart." *Chacruna*. December 17, 2019. https://chacruna.net /why-chronic-microdosing-might-break-your-heart.

Tiwari S. C. "Loneliness: A Disease?" *Indian Journal of Psychiatry* 55, no. 4 (2013): 320–322. https://doi.org/10 .4103/0019-5545.120536.

Totomanova, Iva. "Psychedelics as a Potential Treatment Option in ADHD." Bachelor Thesis. Utrecht University, 2020. https://www.researchgate.net/publication/348277534 _Psychedelics_as_a_Potential_Treatment_Option_in_ADHD.

Toyoda, J. "The Effects of Chlorpromazine and Imipramine on the Human Nocturnal Sleep Electroencephalogram." *Psychiatry and Clinical Neurosciences*, 18 (1964): 198-221. https://doi.org/10.1111/j.1440-1819.1964.tb02384.x.

Tripsafe. "LSD to Shrooms Dosage Converter." *TripsSafe.org*. Accessed May 5, 2021. https://tripsafe.org/lsd-shrooms -dosage-converter/#fn:bad-trip-study.

Tupper, Kenneth W., Evan Wood, Richard Yensen, and Matthew W. Johnson. "Psychedelic Medicine: A Re-emerging Therapeutic Paradigm." *Canadian Medical Association Journal (CMAJ)* 187, no. 14 (2015): 1054–1059. https://doi.org/10.1503/cmaj.141124.

Turner, Erick H., Annette M. Matthews, Efthihia Linardatos, Robert A. Tell, and Robert Rosenthal. "Selective Publication of Antidepressant Trials and Its Influence on Apparent Efficacy." *The New England Journal of Medicine* 358, no. 3 (2008): 252–260. https://doi.org/10.1056/nejmsa065779.

University of California. "Bipolar and Magic Mushroom Study." *Crest.BD*. October 10, 2020. https://www.crestbd .ca/2020/10/10/mushrooms-bipolar-disorder.

Vaidya, V. A., G. J. Marek, G. K. Aghajanian, and R. S. Duman. "5-HT2A Receptor-Mediated Regulation of Brain-Derived Neurotrophic Factor mRNA in the Hippocampus and the Neocortex." *The Journal of Neuroscience* 17, no. 8 (1997): 2785–2795. https://doi.org/10.1523/JNEUROSCI.17-08-02785.1997.

Van Elk, Michiel, George Fejer, Pascal Lempe, Luisa Prochazckova, Martin Kuchar, Katerina Hajkova, and Josephine Marschall. "Effects of Psilocybin Microdosing on Awe and Aesthetic Experiences: A Preregistered Field and Lab-Based Study." *Psychopharmacology (Berlin, Germany)*, (2021). https://doi.org/10.1007/s00213-021-05857-0.

Vann Jones, Simon Andrew, and Allison O'Kelly. "Psychedelics as a Treatment for Alzheimer's Disease Dementia." *Frontiers in Synaptic Neuroscience* 12 (2020): 34. https://doi.org/10 .3389/fnsyn.2020.00034.

Vollenweider, Franz X., and Michael Kometer. "The Neurobiology of Psychedelic Drugs: Implications for the Treatment of Mood Disorders." *Nature Reviews Neuroscience* 11, no. 9 (2010): 642–651. https://doi.org/10.1038/nrn2884.

Vollenweider, Franz X., M. F. Vollenweider-Scherpenhuyzen, A. Bäbler, H. Voge, and Daniel Hell. "Psilocybin Induces Schizophrenia-Like Psychosis in Humans via a Serotonin-2 Agonist Action." *Neuroreport* 9, no. 17 (1998): 3897. https:// doi.org/10.1097/00001756-199812010-00024.

Vollenweider, Franz X., Peter Vontobel, Daniel Hell, and Klaus L. Leenders. "5-HT Modulation of Dopamine Release in

Basal Ganglia in Psilocybin-Induced Psychosis in Man—A PET Study with [11C]raclopride." *Neuropsychopharmacology* 20, no. 5 (1999): 424–433. https://doi.org/10.1016/S0893-133X(98)00108-0.

Voss, Edward W., and Jeffrey L. Winkelhake. "Mechanism of Lysergic Acid Diethylamide Interference with Rabbit Antibody Biosynthesis." *Proceedings of the National Academy of Sciences* 71, no. 4 (1974): 1061–1064. https://doi.org/10.1073/pnas.71.4.1061.

Wacker, Daniel, Sheng Wang, John D. McCorvy, Robin M. Betz, A. J. Venkatakrishnan, Anat Levit, Katherine Lansu, et al. "Crystal Structure of an LSD-Bound Human Serotonin Receptor." *Cell (Cambridge)* 168, no. 3 (2017): 377–389. https://doi.org/10.1016/j.cell.2016.12.033.

Waldman, Ayelet. *A Really Good Day: How Microdosing Made a Mega Difference in My Mood, My Marriage, and My Life.* New York: Alfred A. Knopf, 2017.

Watson, D., L. A. Clark, and A. Tellegen. "Development and Validation of Brief Measures of Positive and Negative Affect: The PANAS Scales." *Journal of Personality and Social Psychology* 54, no. 6 (1988): 1063–1070. https://doi.org/10.1037/0022-3514.54.6.1063.

Webb, Megan, Heith Copes, Peter S. Hendricks. "Narrative Identity, Rationality, and Microdosing Classic Psychedelics." *The International Journal of Drug Policy* 70 (2019): 33–39. https://doi.org/10.1016/j.drugpo.2019.04.013.

Wilcox, James Alex. "Psilocybin and Obsessive Compulsive Disorder." *Journal of Psychoactive Drugs* 46, no. 5 (2014): 393–395. https://doi.org/10.1080/02791072.2014.963754.

Winkelman, Michael J., and Ben Sessa. *Advances in Psychedelic Medicine: State-of-the-Art Therapeutic Applications.* Westport, CT: Praeger, 2019.

Winstock, Adam, Monica Barratt, Jason Ferris, and Larissa Maier. "Global Drug Survey." *Global Drug Survey.* 2017. https://www.globaldrugsurvey.com/wp-content/themes /globaldrugsurvey/results/GDS2017_key-findings-report _final.pdf.

Winter, Gal, Robert A. Hart, Richard P. G. Charlesworth, and Christopher F. Sharpley. "Gut Microbiome and Depression: What We Know and What We Need to Know." *Reviews in the Neurosciences* 29, no. 6 (2018): 629–643.

Wolbach, A. B. Jr., E. J. Miner, H. Isbell. "Comparison of Psilocin with Psilocybin, Mescaline and LSD-25." *Psychopharmacologia* 3 (1962): 219–223. https://doi.org/10 .1007/BF00412109.

Woolley, D. W., and E. Shaw. "A Biochemical and Parhacologi-cal Suggestion about Certain Mental Disorders." *Proceedings of the National Academy of Sciences of the United States of America* 40, no. 4 (1954): 228–31. doi:10.1073/pnas.40.4.228.

Yanakieva, Steliana, Naya Polychroni, Neiloufar Family, Luke T. J. Williams, David P. Luke, and Devin B. Terhune. "The Effects of Microdose LSD on Time Perception: A Randomised, Double-blind, Placebo-Controlled Trial." *Psychopharmacology (Berlin, Germany)* 236, no. 4 (2019): 1159–1170. https://doi.org/10.1007/s00213-018-5119-x.

Zhang, Gongliang, Herborg N. Ásgeirsdóttir, Sarah J. Cohen, Alcira H. Munchow, Mercy P. Barrera, and Robert W. Stackman Jr. "Stimulation of Serotonin 2A Receptors Facilitates Consolidation and Extinction of Fear Memory in C57BL/6J Mice." *Neuropharmacology* 64, no. 1 (2013): 403–413. https://doi.org/10.1016/j.neuropharm.2012.06.007.

Zhuk Olga, Izabela Jasicka-Misiak, Anna Poliwoda, Anastasia Kazakova, Vladlena V. Godovan, Marek Halama, and Piotr P. Wieczorek. "Research on Acute Toxicity and the Behavioral Effects of Methanolic Extract from Psilocybin Mushrooms and Psilocin in Mice." *Toxins* 7, no. 4 (2015): 1018–1029. https://doi.org/10.3390/toxins7041018.

Zimmerman, Mark, Heather L. Clark, Matthew D. Multach, Emily Wash, Lia K. Rosenstein, and Douglas Gazarian. "Symptom Severity and the Generalizability of Antidepressant Efficacy Trials: Changes During the Past 20 Years." *Journal of Clinical Psychopharmacology* 36, no. 2 (2016): 153. https://doi.org/10.1097/JCP.0000000000000466.

ACKNOWLEDGMENTS

First and foremost, I would like to point out that the entirety of this book is a collection of information on various topics within the realm of microdosing, none of which I directly researched. All information is merely collected into a neat and tidy container. That being said, I need to acknowledge all of the authors and their work, cited within.

Research, especially that on psychedelic work, progresses from the previous knowledge gained, and present work "stands on the shoulders of giants."

I would like to personally thank some specific nurses, psychedelic writers/researchers, and pioneers who assisted me in my work. In no particular order: James Fadiman, Torsten Passie, "Spirit Pharmacist" Ben Malcolm, Kelan Thomas, Ido Hartogsohn, Manesh Girn, Balazs Szigeti, Andrew Penn, Aric Mayer, Bryce Koch, Ed Stern, Taraleigh Weathers, Joe Moore, Kyle Buller, Michelle Janikian, Rick Strassman, Beth Weinstein, Ayelet Waldman, Stewart Preston, Daniel Shankin, Carey Clark, and all my previous professors/teachers in school.

ABOUT THE AUTHOR

C. J. Spotswood, MSN, APRN, PMHNP, aka "EntheoNurse," is a board-certified psychiatric mental health nurse practitioner and an integrative behavioral health clinician in a family care clinic. A third-generation male nurse with twenty years of psychiatric nursing experience, he recently completed his Psychiatric Mental Health Nurse Practitioner from the University of Southern Maine. C. J. received his BSN from the University of Maine at Augusta, one of fifteen nursing schools endorsed as a holistic school of nursing, with curricula that included yoga, Reiki, and various other complementary and alternative modalities.

C. J. has been researching and teaching about psychedelics since 2018. He has presented at the American Psychiatric Nurses Association's national conference, taught master classes for Psychedelics Today, and coauthored Psychedelic. Support's continuing education module on psilocybin.

C. J. offers an accredited continuing education program titled "Psychedelics in Psychiatry for Nurses" on his personal website, entheonurse.com. He is a member of OPENurses, the International Association of Psychedelic Nursing, the Psychedelic Medicine Association, and the American Psychiatric Nurses Association. When he is not working, reading, or writing, he can be found exploring Maine's outdoors and craft breweries with his wife, Magen, and his daughter, Malarie.